Our Genetic Future

The Science and Ethics of Genetic Technology

British Medical Association

KU-208-295

Oxford   New York

OXFORD UNIVERSITY PRESS

Oxford University Press, Walton Street, Oxford OX2 6DP

Oxford New York Toronto
Delhi Bombay Calcutta Madras Karachi
Kuala Lumpur Singapore Hong Kong Tokyo
Nairobi Dar es Salaam Cape Town
Melbourne Auckland Madrid

and associated companies in
Berlin Ibadan

Oxford is a trade mark of Oxford University Press

First published 1992 as an Oxford University Press paperback
Reprinted 1992

British Library Cataloguing in Publication Data
Data available

Library of Congress Cataloging in Publication Data
Data available
ISBN 0-19-286156-5

Printed in Great Britain by
J. W. Arrowsmith Ltd, Bristol

Our Genetic Future

The British Medical Association (BMA) is the professional organization representing all doctors in the UK. It was established in 1832 'to promote the medical and allied sciences and to maintain the honour and interests of the medical profession'. The Association advises doctors both collectively and individually on the professional, scientific, and ethical aspects of their work and actions in relation to their patients, colleagues, and society as a whole. In recent years the Association has become increasingly involved in public health. Through the publication of policy statements and in-depth research studies the Association has led the debate on key issues and contributed to the development of better public health policies that affect us all.

In *Our Genetic Future* the Association aims to draw to the attention of health professionals and the public the issues surrounding the impressive developments in genetic research in the past twenty years. The book is the outcome of three years' deliberation by an expert Working Party, with input from the BMA's Board of Science and Education, and Medical Ethics Committee. Scientists, ethicists, and doctors were represented on the Working Party, and further specialist expertise was invited where necessary.

A report from the BMA Professional, Scientific, and International Affairs Division

Project Director	Dr Fleur Fisher
Project Editor	Dr Natalie-Jane Macdonald
Contributing authors	Dr Bernard Dixon
	Dr Erik Millstone
	Dr Robert W. Old
	Mr Simon Shackley
	Ms Henrietta Wallace
Editorial Secretariat	Ms Deborah Pippard
Graphic Designer	Ms Hilary Glanville

The Association is pleased to acknowledge the specialist help provided by Dr Ruth Chadwick, Professor the Reverend Canon Gordon R. Dunstan, Dr David Seedhouse, Mr Anthony Taylor, Professor Sir David Weatherall, Professor Robert Williamson.

PREFACE

The science of genetics is the study of inheritance. In less than a hundred years, the laws governing heredity have been defined and the chemical code in which the units of inheritance is written has been deciphered. In the past twenty years, progress in genetics has been phenomenal and we have gained remarkable insights into the molecular basis of genetic disorders. Developments in genetics are already having practical consequences in clinical medicine, pharmaceutical production, animal experimentation, agriculture, and industry and the potential applications seem limitless. The possibilities and implications of the 'new genetics' are awesome but we lack social and ethical guide-lines to lead us through this uncharted territory. Many people have raised questions about the consequences of applying our new knowledge fearing unwelcome or catastrophic results.

In response to such questions, a resolution was passed at the 1988 Annual Representative Meeting of the British Medical Association (BMA) which recommended that the Association should consider the implications of genetic engineering. Accordingly, a Working Party was established comprised of the following members:

Chairman: Sir Christopher Booth, immediate past Chairman, BMA Board of Science and Education.

Members: Professor D. J. Jeffries, Professor of Virology, the Medical College of St Bartholomew's Hospital, London.

Dr A. W. Macara, Chairman, Representative Body of the BMA and Consultant Senior Lecturer in Epidemiology and Public Health Medicine, University of Bristol.

Dr A. McLaren, Director, Medical Research Council Mammalian Development Unit.

Professor D. B. Morton, Professor of Biomedical Science and Biomedical Ethics, University of Birmingham Medical School.

Colonel M. J. G. Thomas L/RAMC, Member, BMA Board of Science and Education and Commanding Officer, Army Blood Supply Depot.

The Baroness Warnock MA, B.Phil, formerly Mistress of Girton College, Cambridge.

The Working Party met for the first time in early 1989 and agreed that current and future developments in the field of RNA and DNA manipulation should be examined, giving particular consideration to aspects of research and practice which may affect human health and well-being. The Working Party also resolved to develop a framework of ethics to safeguard the community's interest and to consider the need for legislation in areas relating to social and ethical aspects of genetic manipulation. Finally, the Working Party agreed that its findings should be published in a report.

CONTENTS

ABBREVIATIONS AND ACRONYMS

A	Adenine
ACGM	Advisory Committee on Genetic Modification
ACRE	Advisory Committee on Releases to the Environment
BST	Bovine somatotropin
C	Cytosine
cDNA	complementary DNA
CEPH	Centre d'Étude du Polymorphisme Humain
CF	Cystic fibrosis
CVS	Chorionic villus sampling
DMD	Duchenne muscular dystrophy
DNA	Deoxyribonucleic acid
EC	European Community
EPC	European Patent Convention
EPO	European Patent Office
G	Guanine
GMO	Genetically modified organism
HGP	Human genome project
HIV	Human immunodeficiency virus
HSE	Health and Safety Executive
IVF	In vitro fertilization
MRC	Medical Research Council
mRNA	messenger RNA
OECD	Organization for Economic Co-operation and Development
PCR	Polymerase chain reaction
PKU	Phenylketonuria
rDNA	recombinant DNA
RFLP	Restriction fragment length polymorphism
RNA	Ribonucleic acid
tRNA	Transfer RNA
T	Thymine

INTRODUCTION

Genetic and part-genetic diseases affect one in every twenty people by the age of 25 and perhaps as many as two in three people during their lifetime. Developments in the science of genetics offer the possibilities of challenging some of the major causes of illness and premature death in our society, such as heart disease and cancer, as well as a number of uncommon but fatal diseases including muscular dystrophy and cystic fibrosis.

Many common diseases such as coronary artery disease, diabetes, cancer, arthritis, and severe psychiatric disorders have a strong environmental component and the genetic factors do not follow a clear-cut pattern of inheritance. Such diseases result from the exposure of genetically susceptible individuals to environmental causes, and prevention will depend on reducing the levels of exposure either in populations or, more probably, in susceptible individuals. It is most unlikely that we will be able to remove completely the environmental risk factors. Therefore it is important that we learn as much as possible about the genetically determined predisposing factors and hence identify high-risk individuals. The aim is to protect people from the kinds of illnesses to which they are genetically most vulnerable and, where appropriate, to prevent the transmission of the genetic susceptibilities to the next generation. Faster and less costly methods of testing for genetic susceptibility to diseases mean the possibility of population screening for increased risk of these common diseases.

Visions of a new age of genetically informed health care are clouded by doubts and fears of perils which raise, in a new context, familiar issues such as the allocation of resources, the right to privacy, and the protection of confidential information.

The increase in information on an individual's genetic constitution will be beneficial to that person in predicting health risks but could be misused by employers and insurance companies. More accurate and speedy pre-natal diagnosis can be used to prevent children being born with seriously incapacitating disease but could be misused by parents to choose the sex or certain characteristics of their children. These dilemmas do not arise from the information itself but from the uses to which it is put. Serious consideration of these questions by society is therefore vital.

The time is right for discussion regarding how and by whom this emerging genetic knowledge should be used. It is essential that education should be widely available in a way that people can understand and that society as a whole become involved in the decisions about how genetics is to be applied. Already town meetings are being held in the USA to inform people about the Human Genome Project and to solicit opinions on the social and ethical issues that it raises. As well as informing and educating the general public about these issues, doctors and other health care workers require better training in the science and ethics of genetics. The 1990 Royal College of Physicians report on 'Teaching Genetics to Medical Students' revealed much scope and many options for improvement. The average number of hours of timetabled genetics teaching in the clinical courses of UK medical schools is only about five and a half. This is inadequate to cover fully such a complex subject.

There are dangers in large scientific projects. If scientific progress becomes the sole ideal, then the importance of human rights is likely to be diminished or ignored. In relation to genetics, people have voiced fears that mastery and control over our genetic constitution will raise possibilities of **eugenics**. We need to maintain a distinction between diagnosis and treatment of disease and the selection of 'desirable' traits. The ownership and control of genetic information and the issue of consent to use such information must be addressed. Society must deal satisfactorily with the 'test cases'.

Of great concern to many people is that any genetic

information arising out of the molecular research should be used fairly, with respect to insurance, employment, criminal law, and education. People fear that they might be put into high risk or uninsurable groups because of genetic factors. Most medical information pertains only to the individual patient. However, one of the factors peculiar to genetics and which raises particular ethical considerations is that genetic information more often than not is important to the entire genetic family. The very nature of genetic information as something that is shared among family members raises problems over privacy and disclosure.

Normally, regulation of developments in medicine and science follows on from discoveries or inventions, and usually only after public concerns have been raised and public opinion has more or less settled. On matters which are perceived to be of major importance to all people, controls tend not to be left to the scientific or medical communities themselves. For example, embryo research was considered by the government-appointed Warnock Committee and its report formed the foundation for the Human Fertilization and Embryology Act 1990. Similarly, in 1989 the government established a committee, chaired by Sir Cecil Clothier, to consider the ethics of gene therapy. The Committee published its report in January 1992 and the government is expected to act on its recommen- dations in the near future, following a public consultation exercise.

Decisions on the use of genetic modification in one country will increasingly affect other countries as population migration increases. It is therefore imperative that decisions about, for example, germ-line gene therapy take into account opinions of people world-wide. The international co-ordination needed for the Human Genome Project, which will be discussed later, may aid this process but the developing countries need to be adequately represented, especially as they constitute such a large proportion of the world's population.

All too often the debate on the new genetics is conducted in polarized terms, as if it were either an unalloyed blessing or a curse. For supporters, genetic modification presents major opportunities in the development of drugs, screening methods for diseases, and the possibilities of gene therapy. For those opposed, the new genetics appears to be the scientific and medical community interfering with our environment and our inheritance and at times even 'playing God'.

We believe that biotechnology and genetic modification are in themselves morally neutral. It is the uses to which they are put which create dilemmas. The challenge which faces us is to try to achieve an optimal future: one which maximizes the benefits of genetic modification and minimizes the harms.

In the following pages we will take the reader through the science of genetics, from the first experiments of Gregor Mendel with the smooth and wrinkled seeds of edible peas to the very recent application of gene therapy in patients with a severe immune deficiency disease. By using a step-by-step approach together with a comprehensive glossary we hope to help readers new to the subject to come to terms with some of the more complex language and terminology. We will focus not just upon genetics and its possibilities as applied to human beings but also the effects on micro-organisms, plants, and animals. This is first because many of the treatments or investigative techniques which are ultimately used in people have been initially applied and refined in these other species. Secondly, as already mentioned, some of the worries that the rapid developments in genetics raise are related to the possible detrimental effects on our plants and animals—from, for example, the release of genetically modified organisms.

The acquisition of new knowledge in genetics seems to occur at a tremendous pace. During the writing of this book constant revision has had to be undertaken to include new developments. We can therefore only apologize if some readers feel that on occasions we are already out of date. However, the same criticism cannot be levelled at the second part of our report, which looks at the social and ethical implications of the new genetics with which we are all attempting to come to terms. The progress of genetic knowledge, while creating some new ethical dilemmas, seems largely to magnify existing ethical problems in medicine. Many, for example those concerning privacy and disclosure, place long-standing unsolved dilemmas of medical ethics in a new context. As a community, our difficulties are compounded by the fact that no one is yet in a position to forecast accurately either the benefits or the risks from some of the developments of genetic modification.

Our predicament would be a great deal simpler if we could simply ask, in respect of any proposed development, questions such as 'Is it safe?', 'Will it enable us to find cures for genetic diseases?', and 'How much will it cost?', and receive unequivocal answers. Unfortunately life is not so straightforward. The totality of scientific knowledge which we would like to have when making judgements about the future is rarely available. Consequently, the judgements which need to be made, and the decisions which need to be taken, are complex, contestable, and often incomplete. Until we have answers to these questions it is not possible to form settled views about the acceptability of some developments. Where we have been able, we have recommended practices, regulations, or policies which will help to guide the way forward. In other areas, we emphasize the importance of consultation and public discussion into which new information can be fed as it becomes available.

It is not possible to provide any guarantees against, or insurance for, mistakes. It may be extremely unlikely that something will go seriously wrong with genetic modification, but serious errors could be catastrophic. At this stage in the development and application of genetic modification, when we seek to optimize benefits over risks, it is prudent to err on the side of caution and above all to learn from our accumulating experience.

Chapter One

A Quick Overview

> But where the bull and cow are milk-white,
> They never do beget a coal-black calf.

Shakespeare's observation, in *Titus Andronicus*, is one of many attesting to the continuity that is so apparent in the process of heredity. Not only do cows beget cows, rather than horses or kangaroos, they also tend to produce calves that later become adults with colouring and other characteristics which are recognizably the same as those of their parents. So too with human procreation. If two relatively tall people have children, the offspring too will tend to be tall. Buy some nasturtium seeds for your garden, and you will find that the plants tend to resemble those pictured on the packet. The word 'tend' is necessary because, as we also know, not all of the attributes of a particular animal or plant 'breed true' or can be clearly traced from one generation to the next. Mum and dad may be obese, but their baby can grow into an adult of less than average weight. Except in the case of identical twins, siblings often differ one from the other, sometimes dramatically so. Animal breeding may fail to produce the expected results. The photograph on the seed packet can be seriously misleading.

For centuries, enquiring minds have sought to understand both the constancy that is so obvious in the inheritance of characteristics by animals and plants, and also the variability seen in families and the changes that sometimes occur between one generation and the next. They have tried to fathom the answers to two central questions. First, which characteristics are truly inherited and which are influenced by dietary, environmental, and other external factors? What, in other words, are the relative contributions of nature and nurture? Secondly, what are the mechanisms that determine inherited traits—the colour of a flower, for example, or the occurrence of a hereditary disease such as haemophilia in humans? How are characteristics of this sort conveyed from parent to offspring?

In building up our present understanding of heredity, biologists relied initially on simple observations of both the sameness and the variability that is apparent among the profusion of life on earth. In humans, family trees were particularly helpful in bringing out recurrent patterns of inherited qualities. Gradually, however, the mere recording and comparison of such observations was augmented by more practical experience. First came the lessons learned from attempts, initially somewhat haphazard but later of increasing sophistication, to breed domestic and food animals and crop plants with desired qualities. More recently, over the past century, geneticists began to examine the nature of heredity with increasing precision, as they carried out actual experiments spanning the generations. The results have revealed the uncanny accuracy with which specific traits are replicated between one generation and the next, and also the material basis of both sudden and gradual changes when these occur.

Now, with the advent of genetic modification, we have opportunities to alter the hereditary constitution of living things in ways that are both very precise and also distinct from the changes that already occur in nature. These developments have stemmed from successive advances in our understanding of the molecules responsible for inheritance.

When biologists first started practising the science of genetics, they worked with units of heredity—later defined as **genes**. Passed from parent to offspring, these were imagined to be the material carriers of traits such as the colours of human hair and flower petals. But in contrast to, say, the early anatomists poring over the human skeleton, the first geneticists had to study things—genes—that had no known, tangible form. Their existence could only be deduced from the appearance of specific characteristics in offspring following sexual union and in the products of animal and plant breeding.

Decades elapsed before the combined labours of geneticists and others compiled our modern picture of genes. We now know that genes are parts of **chromosomes**, which occur in the nuclei of living cells. They are pieces of **DNA (deoxyribonucleic acid)** which carry in coded form information that determines hereditary traits, just as a musical score contains the instructions for performing a piece of music. Once this, the physical basis of inheritance, was well understood, it became possible to contemplate ways of altering genes artificially for medical, agricultural, and other purposes. That is what genetic modification means.

At the heart of the biological revolution that has facilitated manœuvres of this sort is the science of molecular biology. Based on discoveries made in Cambridge during the 1950s and 1960s, molecular biology focuses on certain very large molecules in living cells—principally proteins and nucleic acids (DNA and the closely related **ribonucleic acid, RNA**). It explains how coded instructions, carried as genes which comprise the DNA double helix, are translated with the help of RNA into specific proteins. Some of these proteins form part of the structure of living cells and tissues. Others are **enzymes** that catalyse particular chemical reactions. Together, they determine the appearance and behaviour of the organisms of which they are part.

Molecular biology accounts for the three cardinal features of heredity. It explains the faithful copying of DNA, and thus of the genes it carries, when cells divide and when the hereditary material is passed forward from one generation to the next. Secondly, it shows how parental genes are shuffled together to produce new combinations as a result of sexual union. Thirdly, it illustrates the emergence of novelty through **mutation**. Errors in the replication process, and other types of alteration in the structure of DNA, are the basis of mutation.

These were the questions—the central riddles of biology—that molecular biologists attacked during the first two or three decades of their new science. Over the past fifteen years, however, molecular biology has ceased to be a purely descriptive activity, a branch of pure science. It has now spawned applications. These are methods of locating and characterizing genes with great accuracy, and of altering them and moving genes from one organism to another. Techniques of this sort have rendered possible the craft of genetic modification.

The earliest gene transfers were conducted in **bacteria** and other **microbes**. As a result, industrial companies are already harnessing genetically modified micro-organisms to manufacture pharmaceutical and other products. Plant genetic modification proved to be more difficult at first, but has now become a practical proposition too. Least advanced at present is animal, including human, genetic modification. Although offering many potential benefits, this type of work poses even greater ethical and practical questions than those generated by genetic modification in microbes and plants.

The safety and ethical implications of genetic modification have already attracted considerable attention in the media. There is even a Desmond Bagley novel (*The Enemy*) focusing on the issue. At least in some countries, much of the public discussion of the issue has been dominated by lobbyists who to one degree or another oppose these new developments. Yet scientists themselves, who were the first to project concerns about possible hazards of genetic modification into the public and political arena, now tend to argue that, given scientific, legal, and ethical controls, most of such work can proceed without significant risk. Scientists have been closely involved in the development of such safeguards and regulations. Now, as this new technology generates increasing numbers of possible benefits in medicine, agriculture, and other fields, it is more essential than ever that future research and development proceed with public understanding and support.

Chapter Two

Life and Heredity

Inheritance of what?

When Charles Darwin's *Origin of Species* appeared in 1859, it was an overnight sensation, triggering considerable controversy, particularly within the Church, because it seemed to discredit the idea of divine creation and the belief that humans are the most important creatures in the natural world. However, popular among both scientists and non-scientists, Darwin's best-seller explained—in outline, but with abundant evidence—a plausible mechanism through which life had evolved on earth. At the centre of evolution, Darwin saw the natural selection of variants that arose spontaneously among populations of animals and plants. A variant with a new trait making it better adapted to a particular environment was more likely to survive and leave progeny than one that was less well adapted.

Because the trait was inherited, the progeny would tend to compete with and supplant, in that environment, those of less well adapted parents. Over aeons of time, many more spontaneous changes would occur. Some would confer a competitive disadvantage and be eliminated. Some would be neutral. But successive changes making the animal or plant better suited to its environment would eventually produce a population so different that its members would no longer be able to cross-fertilize with those in the original population. This, Darwin argued, was the way in which new species arose. At the same time, he believed that there was one serious objection to his scenario. How could evolution proceed in this way, when a favourable change in one individual was certain to be 'diluted' in that organism's progeny and diluted further in subsequent generations? The problem arose in Darwin's mind because he, like other biologists of his day, saw heredity as a blending of parental characteristics. Linked with the ancient, erroneous belief that blood was the carrier of inherited traits, this idea also had respectable supporting evidence. What better explanation, when a tall woman and a short man produce a child of average height, than that the hereditary material has been blended together, like red wine mixed with white?

The real answer to Darwin's difficulty is that inheritance rests not on a fluid that can be diluted down the generations but on discrete units, originally portrayed as particles, that are passed from parents to offspring. The existence and behaviour of these particles explains one particular puzzle—the way in which an inherited trait may lapse in one generation or more and then reappear totally unaltered in a later generation.

The gene—a tangible idea

Around the same time that Darwin's *Origin of Species* was revolutionizing people's perceptions of their place in the natural world, but unknown to the English naturalist, an Augustinian monk in Moravia was conceiving the idea of particulate inheritance and proving its operation. Through a series of meticulously designed experiments, Gregor Mendel saw that inherited characteristics are determined by units of hereditary material which are passed, usually unaltered, down the generations. They have been called genes since the Danish biologist, Wilhelm Johannsen, introduced the term in 1909.

The key experiments, conducted in the monastery garden at Brunn (now Brno, in Czechoslovakia), were those in which Mendel crossed different varieties of edible peas, examined the offspring, and realized that certain traits sometimes eclipsed others. When he crossed tall and short plants, for example, all of the progeny were tall. He thus described tallness as

dominant over shortness. But a cross between two of these tall offspring yielded about a quarter of short peas in the next generation. The hidden, **recessive** gene for shortness had reasserted itself (see Fig. 2.1).

Repeating these crosses hundreds of times, together with other crosses between plants with other pairs of qualities, Mendel saw that the ratios of the progeny became extremely precise. This led him to the simple explanation which is now one of the central tenets of genetics. Every plant (and every animal) carries a 'double dose' of each of its genes. If both members of a pair of genes are dominant, then that trait (for example, tallness in the pea plants) is expressed. It is also expressed if one gene is dominant and the other recessive. But if both genes are recessive, then that trait (shortness in the peas) is expressed instead.

In the pea experiments, these combinations produce an overall ratio of one short to three tall plants. But two out of every three tall plants carry a masked, unexpressed gene for shortness. Although all three possess the same **phenotype** (appearance), two have a **genotype** (genetic make-up) different from the other.

Sometimes, dominance is not complete. Red campions crossed with white campions, for example, produce pink progeny. At first sight, this looks suspiciously like blending inheritance. But if the pink progeny are crossed one with another, there will be an average ratio of one red flower, one white, and two pink in the next generation. Clearly, blending inheritance cannot account for the reappearance of red and white flowers. The true explanation is that the red plants carry two genes for redness, the white flowers two white genes, and the pink flowers one of each. The pink flowers arise because neither of the genes is dominant over the other. With dominance, the 1 : 2 : 1 ratio becomes 3 : 1, as in the case of the tall and short peas.

A more complex ratio came to light when Gregor Mendel studied the inheritance of two pairs of characteristics together, rather than a single pair. In one series of experiments, he

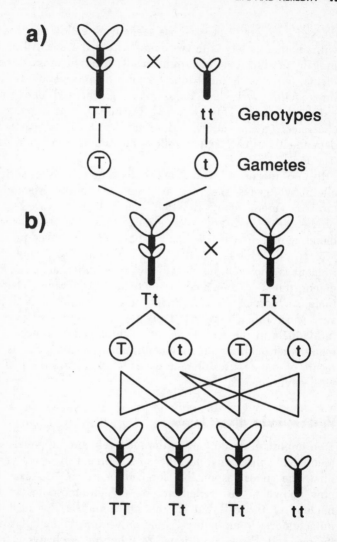

Fig. 2.1 (a) Mendelian cross showing dominance. (b) Cross showing reappearance of recessive gene for shortness in the second generation

Note: in (a) all offspring are tall. In (b) the ratio of phenotypes is three tall plants to one short plant and the ratio of genotypes is 1 : 2 : 1.

crossed a variety of peas whose seeds were yellow and round with another variety with green and wrinkled seeds. All of the progeny produced yellow, round seeds. When he crossed these plants, however, Mendel found a ratio of nine yellow round, three yellow wrinkled, three round green, and one green wrinkled seeds. This occurred because the two pairs of characters (green–yellow and round–wrinkled) segregate independently of each other, yellow and round being dominant (see Fig. 2.2).

By no means all traits are determined by the sort of alternative genes that are apparent in simple Mendelian crosses. Often, many different genes interact together to produce the end-result—an arrangement that mimics the blending inheritance in which most biologists believed prior to Mendel. In contrast to his short and tall peas, height in humans is one example of such **polygenic** inheritance. As first demonstrated by the English mathematician Francis Galton, there is a 'normal curve' for height in the population, with few very short and few very tall people and a bulge of average individuals in the middle. As with intelligence, weight, and many other qualities showing continuous variation, this is the result of numerous different genes working together, along with environmental factors.

What Mendel didn't know

Two important exceptions to the relatively simple patterns of Mendelian inheritance have become apparent in recent years. First, the genes responsible for certain human diseases are now known to be carried not on the chromosomes in the nucleus of the cell but in the mitochondria. Because the mitochondria in an embryo come only from the cytoplasm of the egg cell, these conditions are inherited exclusively from the mother. They include various so-called mitochondrial myopathies, which are characterized by muscular weakness, and Leber's hereditary optic myopathy, which causes blindness. Secondly, research in recent years has shown that the

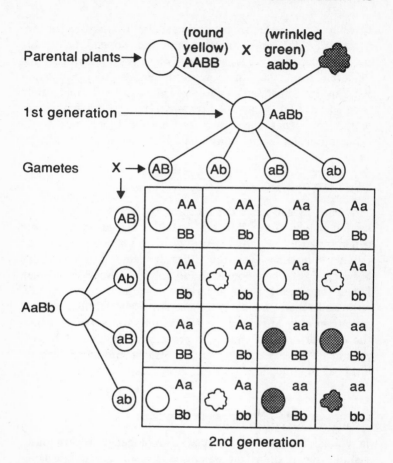

Fig. 2.2 Mendelian cross showing inheritance of two pairs of characteristics

Note: the ratio of the progeny in the second generation: 9 round yellow : 3 wrinkled yellow : 3 round green : 1 wrinkled green.

expression of a gene may vary depending on whether it came from the mother or the father. This is the result of a phenomenon called parental imprinting of genes, the reason for which is not yet fully understood but which could have implications for human disease. For example, it now appears that the same deletion on chromosome 15 may cause two completely different clinical syndromes depending on the parental origin of the gene: in Prader-Willi syndrome the deletion is on the chromosome inherited from the father whereas in Angelman syndrome the deletion is maternally derived. It also seems that parental imprinting of tumour suppressor genes may increase the likelihood of certain cancers developing in individuals receiving such genes.

What is a hybrid?

The word **hybrid** describes the progeny in the sort of crosses carried out by Gregor Mendel. But it is also used in a more general sense for any offspring of genetically dissimilar parents, sometimes even from different species. Mules (hybrids between horses and donkeys) and zebroids (hybrids between horses and zebras) are generally infertile, because of differences in their parents' chromosomes. Hybrids, the results of genetic mixing, are entirely distinct from **chimaeras**, in which the cells of distinct organisms are mixed together. Although natural chimaeras exist, they can also be produced through artificial modification, as with sheep-goat chimaeras.

Chromosomes—the carriers of genes

In animal and plant cells, genes are located in structures, visible under the light microscope, called chromosomes. Humans have twenty-three pairs of chromosomes. A complete set of pairs of genes, carried in a complete set of pairs of chromosomes, is present, as a rule, in every cell. There are a few minor exceptions to this, such as human red blood cells, which contain no nuclei or genes whatever. There is also one other major exception—that of the reproductive cells. Also called **germ cells** or **gametes** (ova and spermatozoa in animals, and their counterparts in plants), these contain only one copy of each gene. A new pairing is established when gametes meet at fertilization. Thus one of the genes in each pair comes from one parent, and the other from the other parent.

Meiosis is the name of the process, occurring during the development of germ cells in the reproductive organs, in which the chromosomes are halved in number from the complete (**diploid**) set to the half (**haploid**) set. **Mitosis** is the corresponding process in all other tissues of the body, when diploid cells divide and their full complement of chromosomes (and thus genes) is copied and maintained. This is what happens during the growth of animal and plant tissues (see Fig. 2.3).

Alternative traits such as tallness and shortness in peas are determined by genes that occupy the same site or **locus** on a particular chromosome. These are called **alleles**. Examples of alleles in people include the genes that are responsible for the ABO and Rhesus blood groups. Although Mendel worked with pairs of characteristics and thus pairs of alleles, many loci have several different alleles specifying alternative characteristics. An animal or plant carrying two identical alleles (for example, a pea plant with two tallness genes) is said to be **homozygous** for that trait. An organism with two different alleles at a particular locus is described as **heterozygous**. This distinction has important medical implications—for example, in sickle cell anaemia. The disease appears in individuals who are homozygous for a gene that produces an abnormal form of **haemoglobin**, which distorts red blood cells and impedes blood circulation. Heterozygotes, whose sickle cell gene is masked by its normal allele, make normal haemoglobin and do not develop sickle cell anaemia, although they can of course pass on the gene to their offspring. The sickle cell allele seems to have been maintained in certain regions of the world, rather than being eliminated during evolution, because heterozygotes enjoy significant protection against malaria—i.e., when malaria is present, carriers are healthier than those who are homozygous 'normal'.

Polymorphism is the name given to the existence in one population of individuals with two or more discrete genotypic

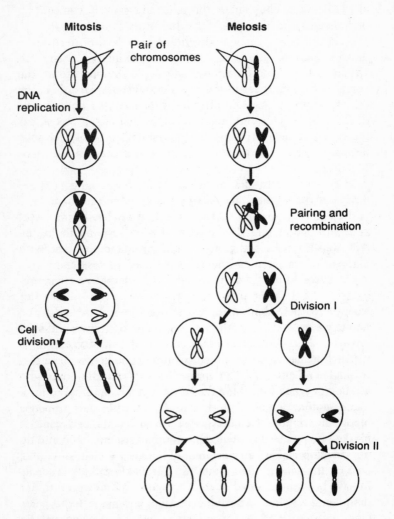

Fig. 2.3 Mitosis and meiosis
Note: recombination during meiosis is shown.

differences. If the mixture has persisted for many generations, it is termed a balanced polymorphism. One example is a population that includes healthy people with normal haemoglobin, healthy people carrying the sickle cell trait, and individuals homozygous for the sickle cell gene.

Mendel died in 1884, but his work did not attract serious attention among biologists until the beginning of this century. Their realization of its significance was heightened by the discovery of chromosomes (so-called after the Greek words for coloured bodies, because they stain strongly with certain dyes) and meiosis. Suddenly, it became clear that many of the observed facts of inheritance could be accounted for on the basis of hereditary particles carried on chromosomes. The American biologist William Sutton was one of the first to make this explicit claim, although the German zoologist August Weismann had suggested as early as the 1880s that 'chromatic loops' (chromosomes) were the hereditary material.

Can acquired characteristics be inherited?

An alternative to Darwin's theory of evolution was that of the French botanist Jean Lamarck. He believed that acquired characteristics—a blacksmith's large biceps, for example—could be passed from parents to offspring. On this theory, the giraffe has evolved a longer and longer neck by continually stretching to reach high branches. August Weismann argued that 'Lamarckism' was impossible because the germ line—the cells that produce eggs and spermatozoa—was separate from the somatic line—the other cells of the body. His views are still considered valid. There is no mechanism through which bodily changes, such as muscular development, can affect the messages carried from one generation to the next through the genes.

Charting the genes

The next major step forward came between 1910 and 1919, when the American geneticist Thomas Hunt Morgan recognized that, in contrast to the independent segregation reflected in the 9 : 3 : 3 : 1 ratio studied by Mendel, many characters tend to be inherited together. The explanation of this, called **linkage**, provides an immediate, practical connection between the work of the pioneers of genetics and the efforts now going into the mapping of the genes on the human chromosomes.

Instead of using plants, Morgan decided to work with the fruit fly *Drosophila*, which had several advantages for genetic research. The flies are easy to breed and grow, and possess only four pairs of chromosomes. They also have a life cycle of just fourteen days, which facilitates the rapid tracing of characteristics from one generation to the next. Initially sceptical about Mendel's work, Morgan soon confirmed the existence of Mendelian ratios in the offspring of *Drosophila*. He then found that in certain crosses certain genes remained linked together more frequently than would be expected if they were randomly assorted. Once Morgan had spotted that there were four groups of linked genes, the explanation was compelling: *Drosophila* had four linkage groups because the genes were linked together on the four chromosomes.

The most obvious example of linkage concerns the sex chromosomes. In most vertebrate animals, many invertebrates and some plants, the female has two X chromosomes and the male one X and one Y chromosome. In birds, butterflies, moths, and some fish, males are XX and females XY. These chromosomes not only determine sex; they carry genes for other traits too. Red-green colour blindness in humans, for example, is determined by a recessive gene on the X chromosome. The condition is thus commoner in men. But the gene is carried by women who do not suffer from its effects because it is masked by a dominant gene conferring normal colour vision. Other **X-linked** diseases include haemophilia and Duchenne muscular dystrophy.

In his experiments with *Drosophila*, Thomas Hunt Morgan found that even traits on the same chromosome became reassorted. Although this did not happen frequently, he began to suspect that chromosomes could break and then recombine during meiosis and mitosis. This led him to a 'thought experiment', based on the greater chance of a break occurring between two genes that were far apart on a chromosome than between two that were close together. If this were so, the frequency with which genes were reassorted might be used as a measure of the distance between them. Crossing fruit flies carrying many different traits, Morgan then showed that he was right. The end-result was a series of maps showing the linear order of genes on the chromosomes of *Drosophila*.

Mutation—the source of novelty

Like the shuffling of a pack of cards, the reassortment of genes clearly generates novelty in the form of new combinations. But what is the origin of those entirely new genes upon which natural selection operates, according to Darwin's theory of evolution? The scientist who first answered this question was one of Morgan's students, Hermann J. Muller. He found that genes (which were increasingly being portrayed as analogous to beads on a string) could be induced to transform, or mutate, into genes coding for a significantly different trait. By bombarding *Drosophila* with powerful doses of X-rays, Muller altered genes responsible for characteristics such as eye colour, body bristles, and wing shape, thereby producing flies with unusual and in some cases bizarre traits.

Muller had encountered some of these mutations previously in natural populations of fruit flies. But irradiation increased their frequency by a factor of 15,000 or more. Other mutations (for example, 'splotched wing' and 'sex-combness') Muller had never seen before. These developments showed that despite the permanency and faithful copying of genes which were responsible for the results observed by Gregor Mendel, units of heredity *could* be altered. A few mutations prove beneficial to the organism concerned. They form the raw material for evolutionary change and improvement. Most mutations are harmful, many being quickly eliminated because they place the plant, animal, or microbe carrying them at a severe disadvantage in a particular environment. We shall discuss the molecular basis of mutation later.

All humans, like other animals, carry potentially dangerous and even lethal mutant genes. These are not expressed because they are recessives, masked by normal dominant genes. The chances of two such genes coming together are increased greatly when very closely related individuals reproduce, as in an incestuous relationship. This is the biological basis of laws proscribing inbreeding between close relatives.

The importance of sex

Mutations in **somatic cells** (for example, those responsible for patches of skin of different texture and pigmentation on the back of your hand) are not inherited. But those occurring in germ cells provide the raw material for evolution by natural selection. Equally important is the generation of new combinations of genes during sexual union. First, pairs of chromosomes come close together during meiosis. Each one splits into two **chromatids** and material is then randomly exchanged between the paternal and maternal chromosomes. Mutations (including deletions of genetic material) may occur during this **crossing over** or **recombination**. Secondly, chromosomes are reassorted during meiosis, each gamete receiving a set randomly composed of paternal and maternal chromosomes. Even with just four pairs of chromosomes, sixteen different combinations are possible in the gametes. Finally, sexual union gives rise to 256 (16 × 16) possible combinations of chromosomes in the offspring of two parents.

The chemistry and chemicals of life

Towards the end of the 1800s and during the early decades of this century, in parallel with the development of what we now term genetics, scientists were creating another new discipline, biochemistry, as they probed the chemical processes associated

with living organisms. Their first discoveries (which began to
demolish vitalism, the idea that life could not be explained on
the basis of chemistry and physics alone) concerned chemical
conversions achieved by relatively simple organisms. In
Germany, for example, Eduard and Hans Buchner found that a
non-living, cell-free extract of yeast could ferment sugar to
alcohol. Formerly this process was thought to depend on the
yeast being alive. Gradually, it became clear that fermentation
itself was a complex process. The conversion of sugar to
alcohol and carbon dioxide took place in a sequence of steps,
now described as a metabolic pathway. Each step in the
pathway was effected by a natural catalyst known as an
enzyme. Charting the successive stages, with their inter-
mediary products, biochemists eventually constructed a metabolic map—a diagrammatic representation of the overall
transformation, conducted by yeast cells as their means of
obtaining energy.

We now know that living cells are characterized by many
different metabolic pathways. Some, like that of yeast fermentation, bring about the breakdown of food materials. Others
operate to build up the structure of cells and other materials
from simpler substances. The former produce both the energy
and materials that are used as building blocks in the latter.

Not all organisms can promote all of these chains of
transformation. Animal cells, for example, do not ferment
sugar by the process seen in yeasts and many other microbes.
They attack sugar through another metabolic pathway, one that
differs from fermentation in requiring oxygen. When respira-
tion is impaired, animal cells also have a limited capacity to
secure energy by converting sugar to lactic acid in the absence
of oxygen. This is why runners towards the end of a marathon
may experience pain and difficulties in moving, as lactic acid
accumulates in their leg muscles.

Clearly, the metabolic pathways responsible for synthesizing
cellular materials also differ between different types of
organism. Whereas humans and other vertebrates produce
bone and other structural materials, plants synthesize different

'backbones' such as cellulose and lignin. One metabolic pathway unique to green plants is that responsible for photosynthesis, the process through which they harness the energy of sunlight to 'fix' carbon dioxide from the air and thereby produce sugars.

There are four major classes of organic molecules in all living things—carbohydrates, lipids, amino acids, and nucleotides. Carbohydrates consist of glucose and other simple sugars; sucrose and other larger sugar molecules formed by the combination of the simple sugars; and much more complex polysaccharides, such as starch in plants and glycogen in animals, that consist of large numbers of sugar molecules linked together. Sugars are broken down to release energy, while starch and glycogen serve as energy stores. Carbohydrates have other functions too, some of them acting as building materials. Cellulose, the principal construction material of plants, and chitin, which forms the outer casing of insects' bodies, are polysaccharides.

Lipids are sometimes defined as oils, fats, and waxes that are found in living tissues and are insoluble in water. In more precise terms, two particular types of lipids are of special importance. Fatty acids are composed of molecules, one end of which is insoluble in water and the other end of which is water-soluble. They too store energy, but also appear, as phospholipids, in the membranes surrounding cells. Steroids, a further group of lipids, include another component of cell membranes, cholesterol, hormones such as testosterone and cortisone, and vitamin D, which helps to incorporate calcium into bones.

Amino acids are the building blocks of proteins. Almost all proteins, which are very large molecules, are made from a basic set of just twenty amino acids. The particular sequence of amino acids in a protein, and the way the molecule is folded into a complex three-dimensional shape as a result of this sequence, determine its nature and activity. Different types of protein function as enzymes, catalysing biochemical conversions; as immunoglobulins (**antibodies**) that fight infection;

and, in the form of haemoglobin and myoglobin, as transporters and storers of oxygen. Other proteins form structural materials such as muscle, hair, and skin.

Nucleotides are the building blocks of nucleic acids, which carry genetic messages in coded form, and which we shall be considering in detail in Chapter 3. It is the information encoded in one of the nucleic acids, DNA, processed via RNA, that determines the corresponding structures of proteins. Like proteins, nucleic acids are thus very large molecules. They are known as macromolecules (although this term is also used to describe most polysaccharides, which are built out of many smaller building blocks but do not convey hereditary information.)

Cells—the factories of life

The fundamental units of all living things, cells, vary considerably in size. Bacteria have diameters of 1–2 μm (1–2 millionths of a metre), while most animal and plant cells measure about 10 μm. Certain specialized cells are much larger still. Yet their basic construction is remarkably similar, with a thin, flexible membrane (strengthened by an outer, rigid cell wall in plants and microbes) enclosing other structures and chemical activities within the cytoplasm. The cell membrane is not simply a passive container. It plays an active role in regulating the intake of nutrients and the passage of waste products out of the cell.

A key distinction is between **prokaryotes** and **eukaryotes**. Bacteria are prokaryotes. They have no obvious internal organization, such as a nucleus or chromosomes that go through mitosis or meiosis. Usually consisting of single cells, they reproduce simply by dividing and are thought to resemble the primitive organisms seen during the first two billion years of life on earth. Many bacteria carry DNA not only in their primitive 'nucleus' but also in separate **plasmids**. These are small, double-stranded circular DNA molecules, which can reproduce themselves inside the bacterium independently of the main bacterial DNA. They often carry genes that are not absolutely essential for life.

Humans and other animals, plants, insects, fungi, and yeasts are eukaryotes (from the Greek for *true nucleus*). They are usually multicellular, with different groups of cells forming tissues that perform particular functions—for example, the brain in animals and green leaves in flowering plants. Eukaryotes have a nucleus which, like the cell itself, is surrounded by a membrane. So too are other organelles, whose existence ensures that specialized biochemical reactions occur at different sites in the cell. Chloroplasts are organelles in which photosynthesis takes place in plant cells. Mitochondria, which occur in all eukaryotes, are self-replicating organelles within which energy is generated for the cellular economy. Both mitochondria and chloroplasts contain their own DNA, carrying some of the information required for their specialized functions. Ribosomes are the sites at which proteins are synthesized in both eukaryotes and prokaryotes.

How genes determine the chemistry of life

In 1908 an English doctor, Sir Archibald Garrod, drew attention to certain disorders of bodily metabolism that were clearly visible and instantly recognizable. Two examples were albinism, in which the albino individual lacks pigment in the skin and eyes, and alkaptonuria, in which the urine turns dark on standing. Garrod highlighted three striking features of such conditions. They tended to be familial and were commonest among the offspring of cousin marriages. They became apparent in the first days or weeks of life and they were relatively benign and compatible with a normal life expectancy. Garrod suggested that these conditions were attributable to blocks in metabolic pathways, caused by abnormalities in particular genes. If, for example, a sequence of enzymes normally converted substance A successively to B, C, and D, then the failure of any one of those enzymes would have two effects. The substance awaiting transformation would accumulate and there would be a severe shortage of the substance to which it was normally converted. Either of these defects could cause the sort of outward effects observed in what Garrod called 'inborn errors of metabolism'.

Today, one of the best-known examples of a genetically determined condition is phenylketonuria (PKU), in which the amino acid phenylalanine is not converted to tyrosine but accumulates in the blood instead. Unless PKU is prevented by use of a diet free of phenylalanine, the amino acid accumulates in the body and adversely affects the brain, causing mental deficiency.

There was little hard genetic evidence to support Garrod's ideas, which were well ahead of their time. But they have proved essentially correct. During the 1930s US geneticist George Beadle and biochemist Edward Tatum clearly established that the action of particular enzymes could be attributed to specific genes. They studied the mould *Neurospora crassa*, which normally grows in a medium containing glucose, salts, and the vitamin biotin. When Beadle and Tatum irradiated large numbers of *N. crassa* spores, they found one that could grow only if vitamin B_1 was incorporated in the medium, and another that grew only when vitamin B_6 was added instead. This indicated that irradiation had somehow knocked out two different genes and thus their corresponding enzymes in the two organisms, making them dependent on particular nutrients.

Building on Beadle and Tatum's 'one gene–one enzyme' concept, later researchers have established that every gene (with one or two exceptions) determines the structure of one particular protein. This is the key to the relationship between heredity and biochemistry in animals, plants, and microbes. The relationship holds true whether the gene and its corresponding enzyme have long existed or have come from a recent mutation. It also neatly explains the nature of the changes which geneticists wish to make to living organisms.

Chapter Three

Molecular Biology

DNA—the real stuff of inheritance

By the early years of this century, chromosomes were known to contain both DNA (deoxyribonucleic acid) and protein. The DNA appeared to be a relatively simple substance, and to vary little between one species of life and another. Proteins, however, were huge molecules, made up of large numbers of twenty different amino acids. The conclusion seemed obvious. Only proteins had the capacity to carry, in coded form, the vast amount of information needed to specify hereditary traits.

An English bacteriologist, Fred Griffith, and an American chemist, Oswald Avery, were principally responsible for demolishing this piece of conventional wisdom. Working for the Ministry of Health in London during the 1920s, Griffith found that virulent strains of *pneumococci* (bacteria that cause pneumonia in both humans and mice) formed smooth colonies when grown on nutrient agar, whereas non-virulent strains produced rough colonies. Both types were killed by heating. But when Griffith inoculated mice with a mixture of killed smooth bacteria (virulent) and living rough bacteria (non-virulent), the animals developed pneumonia and died. Pneumococci isolated from the diseased mice were the smooth, virulent sort, and remained so when cultured further. This was, therefore, a permanent, heritable change.

Clearly, *something* had been transferred from the killed *pneumococci* and had altered the genetic material in the living bacteria, making them virulent. Oswald Avery, working with Maclyn McCarty and Colin MacLeod at the Rockefeller

Institute in New York during the 1940s, identified the 'something' as DNA. First, they discovered that they could achieve such transformation, as demonstrated by Griffith in mice, simply by growing living rough pneumococci in the presence of killed smooth bacteria. They then purified what they called the transforming principle and found that it was 99.98 per cent DNA. For a while, sceptics continued to believe that the remaining 0.02 per cent protein was really responsible for the alteration in virulence. Most were convinced, however, when Avery and his colleagues demonstrated that DNAase, an enzyme that destroys DNA, prevented transformation.

The DNA molecule contains phosphate, deoxyribose (a sugar), and four substances known as bases—adenine (A), guanine (G), cytosine (C), and thymine (T). Until the late 1940s, a strong argument against the role of DNA as the carrier of hereditary messages was that the bases seemed to occur in equal amounts in all organisms. Using better analytical techniques, however, the Czech-American biochemist Erwin Chargaff demonstrated that the base composition varied enormously in different species. This finding demolished the long-standing belief that the DNA molecule consisted simply of a monotonous repetition of the four bases, one after the other. It indicated instead that the structures of DNA could be complex enough to hold coded messages. The possibility that it was the carrier of such genetic information became stronger when Chargaff found that the composition of DNA in the cells of a particular species was fixed and constant. Three questions remained to be answered. How were the bases, phosphate and deoxyribose, linked together? How was the DNA structure replicated? What was the nature of the code?

X-rays, model building, and the double helix

The technique that provided the key to answering these questions was X-ray diffraction, developed at the Cavendish Laboratory, Cambridge, by Sir William Bragg and his son Sir Lawrence Bragg. A beam of X-rays passes through a crystal, interacts with its atoms, and emerges as a pattern which, captured on film, can be analysed to reveal the structure of the substance in the crystal. During the 1940s another Cambridge scientist, the Austrian-born chemist Max Perutz, began to apply this method to proteins, and in 1953 he demonstrated the structure of haemoglobin. His colleague John Kendrew had a similar success with myoglobin. Together with studies on DNA and RNA, this work marked the advent of molecular biology—the investigation of the structure and behaviour of the macromolecules upon which life depends.

An American biologist, James Watson, and the English physicist Francis Crick deduced the structure of DNA. They used X-ray pictures produced at King's College, London, by the chemist Rosalind Franklin and the physicist Maurice Wilkins, but proceeded largely by imagining possible structures, building models, and then seeing if the model fitted the experimental data. In 1953, after several false trails, they put forward the double helix, which neatly explained how genetic information could be both stored and replicated.

In the centre of the DNA molecule is a helix with two complementary strands of bases running parallel but in opposite directions. The strands are held together by bonds between the bases—adenine always pairing with thymine, and cytosine always pairing with guanine. On the outside of the strands are 'backbones' consisting of phosphate and deoxyribose. The molecule thus consists of a sequence of nucleotides (base linked to a sugar linked to phosphate) (see Fig. 3.1).

The code of life

Just as the dots and dashes of the morse code signify letters of the alphabet, so the order of bases in DNA specifies the sequence of amino acids in proteins. A particular gene—a particular segment of DNA—determines the corresponding structure of a specific protein (or part of a protein). Francis Crick, working in Cambridge with Sydney Brenner, established that a set of three bases specifies each amino acid. In other

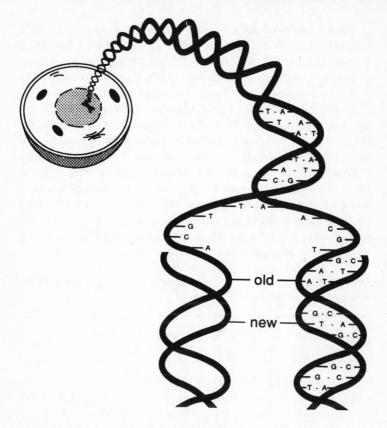

Fig. 3.1 The double helix and DNA replication

words, the coded information in a DNA sequence has to be read
in successive groups of three bases. TGT, for example, codes for
threonine and GTG for histidine. Like any other message, a DNA
strand must be read in one particular direction.

Four different bases, taken three at a time, provide for
$4 \times 4 \times 4 = 64$ possible permutations. That is more than
enough to specify the twenty amino acids found in protein. In
fact, sixty-one of them have been assigned to one amino acid or

another. Threonine, for example, is coded for not only by TGT but also by TGA, TGG, and TGC. The three remaining permutations (ACT, ATT, and ATC) are signals to stop protein production, like full-stops at the end of a sentence (see Table 3.1). The first amino acid produced is always methionine (even if it is eliminated later), so the methionine triplet (TAC) is the starting signal. Except for a slight variation in mitochondria, the code is universal. All organisms, from humans and hippopotami to buttercups and bacteria, use the same system.

There is usually only one correct reading frame for a particular genetic sequence. This can be put out of phase if bases are removed or extra bases added. The result is one type of mutation—a frame-shift mutation, which results in the production of a defective protein that is incapable of playing its normal role in the cell (see Fig. 3.2).

Table 3.1 The genetic code. The abbreviations represent the different amino acids specified by the code.

First position	Second position				Third position
	A	G	T	C	
A	Phe	Ser	Tyr	Cys	A
	Phe	Ser	Tyr	Cys	G
	Leu	Ser	Stop	Stop	T
	Leu	Ser	Stop	Trp	C
G	Leu	Pro	His	Arg	A
	Leu	Pro	His	Arg	G
	Leu	Pro	Gln	Arg	T
	Leu	Pro	Gln	Arg	C
T	Ile	Thr	Asn	Ser	A
	Ile	Thr	Asn	Ser	G
	Ile	Thr	Lys	Arg	T
	Met	Thr	Lys	Arg	C
C	Val	Ala	Asp	Gly	A
	Val	Ala	Asp	Gly	G
	Val	Ala	Glu	Gly	T
	Val	Ala	Glu	Gly	C

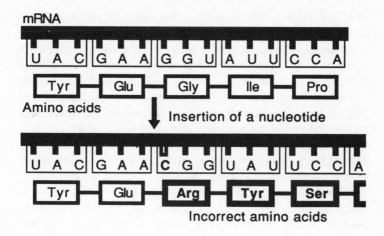

Fig. 3.2 A frame-shift mutation

Turning messages into actions

The DNA double helix, with its coded messages and stop and start signals, comprises the library of genetic information required by a particular animal, plant, or microbe. Wound tightly round itself as 'supercoils', most of the DNA is organized as chromosomes, which are linear in animal and plant cells but circular in bacteria. Converting the information encoded in DNA into proteins requires a second type of nucleic acid—ribonucleic acid (RNA), which is single-stranded and has the sugar ribose instead of the closely related deoxyribose and the base uracil (U) instead of thymine.

When a particular protein is to be produced according to its genetic 'blueprint', the double helix untwists at the appropriate point and the two strands separate. An enzyme, RNA polymerase, then binds to one of the strands—the so-called coding strand. Moving along one base at a time, the enzyme matches each one with a new complementary RNA building block which it then links into a growing chain of **messenger RNA (mRNA)**. This is known as **transcription** (see Fig. 3.3).

The sequences of three consecutive bases in mRNA which code for amino acids are called **codons**.

Messenger RNA is a mobile copy of the corresponding DNA message. Each piece of mRNA passes out through the nuclear membrane and moves to a convoluted membrane called the endoplasmic reticulum, where **translation** takes place (see Fig. 3.3). Ribosomes (which themselves consist of RNA and protein) translate the message into a protein. To do so, they require a third type of RNA known as **transfer RNA (tRNA)**. Each tRNA molecule carries a particular amino acid, together with a corresponding **anticodon** loop, a short piece of RNA that binds with a particular mRNA codon.

The ribosome serves as a jig to bring the appropriate tRNAs together. When two tRNA anticodons become attached to two adjacent mRNA codons, their amino acids also come close, ready to join as part of a protein. The ribosome passes along the mRNA one codon at a time, adding successive amino acids to the chain, until it arrives at a stop signal. The ribosome may then have completed its work, or it may continue through a non-coding region until it finds a start signal for another meaningful sequence. Several ribosomes can move along the same mRNA molecule, each generating the same protein. In bacteria, which have no nuclear membrane to be negotiated by mRNA, transcription and translation occur almost simultaneously.

As well as satisfying the evidence from X-ray diffraction and chemical studies, Watson and Crick's double helix offered an elegant solution to the problem of DNA replication, that is, how hereditary messages are copied from one cell or generation to the next. Clearly, the two complementary strands could untwist, separate, and each attract the necessary building blocks to construct a new partner (see Fig. 3.1). We now know that this is precisely how DNA replicates. First, enzymes called gyrases unwind the two strands. Then other enzymes, DNA polymerases, add the necessary building blocks to re-create each of the complementary strands and re-establish the double helix.

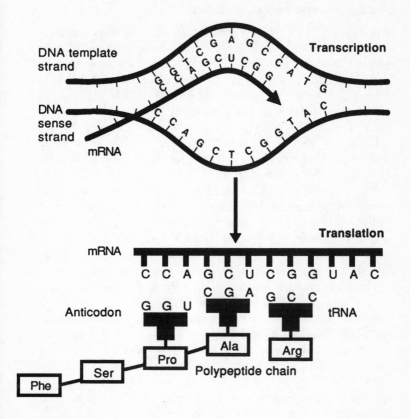

Fig. 3.3 Protein synthesis by transcription and translation

A dogma—and two exceptions

According to the central dogma of molecular biology, information can flow only in one direction—from DNA to RNA to protein. It also passes from DNA to DNA during replication, and from RNA to RNA in certain **viruses** that have (double-stranded) RNA as their genetic material. But the information in proteins is never translated back into DNA or RNA. This accords with the belief that acquired characteristics are not inherited. If they were, then there would have to be some mechanism whereby such characteristics cause heritable changes in the structure of DNA.

There is one important exception to the central dogma. It occurs in certain animal viruses, whose genetic material is RNA. When they infect their host, these **retroviruses** are able to make a DNA copy from their RNA template. The enzyme responsible for this phenomenon, called **reverse transcriptase**, has several potential applications in genetic modification.

There are growing suspicions that there may be exceptions to the rule that all life is based on nucleic acids. Certain diseases that cause slow degeneration of the nervous system, including Creutzfeldt-Jacob disease in humans and scrapie in sheep, seem to be caused by infectious particles that consist of little more than a protein. If these **prions** do contain DNA or RNA, then it must be a very tiny quantity and/or be of unusually small length. Yet they are capable, in an analogous fashion to viruses, of triggering the production of new prion particles in infected cells. Another puzzle is that DNA in healthy tissues carries sequences coding for prion protein. Although by no means proven, it is possible that bovine spongiform encephalopathy (BSE), the so-called 'mad cow disease' that first came to light among British cattle in 1986, is caused by a prion.

Regulation inside the living cell

What is it that prevents all of the genes in a cell from producing their proteins at a maximum rate all of the time?

The answer is that in addition to the genes specifying proteins, which are called structural genes, DNA also contains genes that act as switches. They turn the structural genes on and off as required. Our knowledge of these genes stemmed from research on a bacterium that is capable of living on either glucose or lactose (milk sugar). The organism produces two enzymes, one to ferry lactose into the cell and the other to digest it—but it does so only when lactose is present in the environment. In the absence of lactose, the genes coding for those two enzymes are switched off by a repressor. The repressor sits on an operator, adjacent to the two structural genes, and thus prevents RNA polymerase from transcribing the appropriate messages. Lactose (acting as an inducer) removes the repression. The genes are then translated, and the two enzymes produced, allowing the bacterium to digest lactose. There are many similar examples of gene regulation. A group of adjacent structural genes (often those coding for the successive steps in a particular metabolic pathway) together with their common operator is called an **operon**.

While microbes need to be able to turn certain genes on and off in response to changes in the environment, this is not generally true of animal cells, which have stable surroundings composed of other tissues and body fluids. So although the cells in tissues such as skin, muscle, and nerve all contain the same DNA in their chromosomes, only those genes needed for their specialized functions are translated into enzymes and other proteins. Genes not required are not actually lost as different types of cell differentiate from the original fertilized egg cell. They are simply not expressed. Thus a skin cell does not begin to behave as a liver cell, or vice versa. A partial exception to this rule is the disorderly growth of a tumour, when normal control mechanisms no longer operate.

Nonsense and duplication of effort

Although we think of microbes as primitive organisms, compared with animals and plants, so-called higher organisms do not have their genes organized as economically as one might expect, in highly efficient operons dedicated to specific pathways. Often, the genes for related functions are scattered around on different chromosomes, each being regulated and expressed individually. Another surprise is that a substantial amount of DNA (about 90 per cent in human cells) has no known purpose. It is sometimes termed 'nonsense' or 'junk' DNA, although that which occurs between genes often contains pseudogenes—relics of genes which, like bodily parts such as the vermiform appendix, no longer serve a useful purpose. Presumably some of this DNA really is junk. Otherwise how to explain that the cells of certain salamanders, for example, have twenty times as much DNA as human cells?

Introns are non-coding sequences that occur *within* active genes in animals and plants. These are read during transcription, but pieces of mRNA coding for them are then excised to create a continuous meaningful message. Portions of DNA containing coding information are termed **exons** (see Fig. 3.4). Most higher organisms also contain 'redundant' DNA. This consists of short sequences that are repeated hundreds of times. Some of this DNA may be involved in controlling the activities of chromosomes, but much of it is probably genuine junk. The total genetic material of a particular organism is known as its **genome**.

Duplication of genes, which may appear wasteful or redundant at first sight, can serve a real purpose. Animal and plant DNA, for example, carries many identical genes responsible for the production of the protein found in ribosomes. This is simply a reflection of the need for large numbers of ribosomes for translation. Some apparent repetition has turned out to reflect distinct but closely related proteins. For example, human and other mammalian cells contain several genes coding for haemoglobin. Some of these produce adult haemoglobin and others fetal haemoglobin—a molecule whose slightly different structure reflects its role of carrying oxygen in the womb. The appropriate genes are switched on and off at the appropriate time.

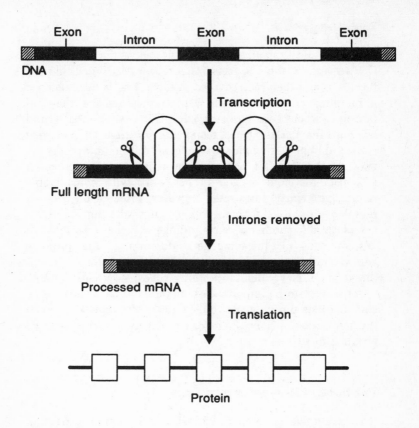

Fig. 3.4 Processing messenger RNA

Jumping genes

One of the most remarkable discoveries about the behaviour of
DNA, made by the US geneticist Barbara McClintock during
the 1940s and then rediscovered in the 1970s, is the existence
of jumping genes. McClintock was studying maize at the Cold
Spring Harbor Laboratory in the USA when she found
evidence that certain genes, responsible for traits such as seed
colour, jumped spontaneously from one chromosome to
another. But this did not occur by crossing-over, and other
biologists therefore reacted to her work with considerable
scepticism. Thirty years later, however, research on bacteria
revealed virtually the same phenomenon—the jumping from
one plasmid to another of genes coding resistance to antibiotics.
We now know that the actual genes do not jump; they produce
copies of themselves which are then inserted at other points in
the genome. Nevertheless, jumping genes, now called transposons, seem to be important as another source of novel gene
combinations during evolution. In 1983, McClintock received
the first unshared Nobel Prize for Physiology or Medicine to be
awarded to a woman.

The book of life—with misprints

It is instructive to compare biological information, carried in
nucleic acids and proteins, with the written words of a book.
The book of the human genome, for example, can be thought of
as consisting of two sets of twenty-three volumes, representing
the twenty-three pairs of homologous chromosomes in the
nucleus of human cells. The average volume has about 2,000
loose-leaf pages, one for each gene. These may occur in small
chapters containing related genes that are next to each other on
the chromosome. The complete set of volumes passed on by
one parent to a child contains an arbitrary combination of the
volumes received from that parent's mother and father, with
some recombination of the loose-leaf pages within each

volume. Thus a particular volume that is passed on may contain sections derived from one parent interspersed with sections from the other.

The analogy continues in the coded form of information—as letters, combined as words, in a printed communication; and as bases combined as genes, in the living cell. The exact replication of DNA when cells divide is reflected in the copying of a printed work by a scribe or typesetter. And the translation of base sequences into amino acid sequences is not unlike the translation of one written language into another. In both copying and translation, errors (mutations) can arise. Even the literary activity of editing has a parallel in the living cell, as when a nonsense sequence, faithfully copied during transcription, is edited out before mRNA passes through the nuclear membrane for translation by ribosomes.

Sequencing genes and proteins

Molecular biology, and its application in genetic modification, is essentially concerned with information—messages carried in nucleic acids, which are translated precisely into the structures of equally complex enzymes and other proteins. The sequencing of the amino acids in proteins, and bases in nucleic acids, is thus of paramount importance. The first person to work out the complete amino acid sequence of a protein was the English biochemist Fred Sanger, also working in Cambridge during the 1950s. He used a digestive enzyme, trypsin, to break down a highly complex molecule, the hormone insulin, into small fragments. He then separated these constituents by using chromatography (in which molecules of different sizes migrate at different rates across a sheet of paper, one edge of which is dipped into a solvent) and **electrophoresis** (in which migration is promoted by an electric current). Thirdly, Sanger determined their amino acid sequences, before reassembling the short fragments into longer ones and deducing the structure of the complete molecule.

Sanger's work was highly innovative—he won a Nobel Prize

in 1958, four years before Watson, Crick and Wilkins, and Perutz and Kendrew, received the same accolade for their work on the structures of DNA and proteins respectively. But it was also extremely painstaking work. Today, protein sequencing is an automated procedure. Machines are now capable of determining the order of hundreds of amino acids in a single day. Databases have been established around the world to hold both the sequences and the three-dimensional structures of thousands of different proteins. This information can be displayed on computer terminals, allowing researchers to study the detailed shape of molecules, and to consider changes designed to alter the behaviour of an enzyme or other protein.

Electrophoresis can also be used to determine the base sequences of DNA. One approach is to separate the two strands of the double helix and insert a radioactive phosphate molecule at one end of a single-stranded fragment. The labelled DNA is then divided into four batches, each of which is given a different treatment to break the chain immediately before one of the four different bases. The fragment lengths are then compared by electrophoresis. If, for example, cleavage before adenine bases produces fragments with 6, 9, and 15 bases, then adenine must occur at positions 7, 10, and 16. Putting all four patterns together reveals the complete sequence of bases (see Fig. 3.5). As with proteins, automated sequencing machines have been introduced, and data-banks now carry the sequences of thousands of genes and of longer pieces of DNA such as plasmids. The entire genomes of certain viruses have been determined, and there are future plans to sequence the whole of the human genome.

Sex among the microbes

As we saw earlier, sexual reproduction is an extremely important mechanism for generating genetic diversity. Evolution would be exceedingly slow if spontaneous, random mutation was the only source of novelty. But what takes the place of sex in microbes such as bacteria? The answer—a

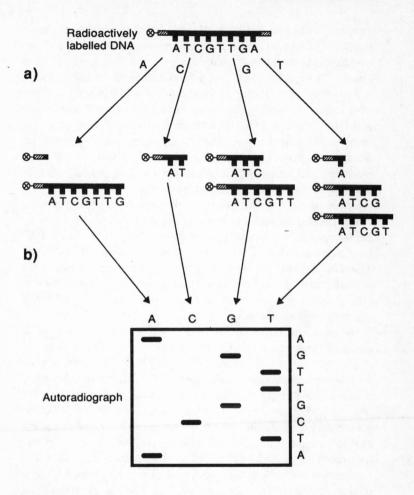

Fig. 3.5 DNA sequencing

Note: in (a) the radioactive DNA is divided into 4 batches and each is treated to break the DNA immediately before one of the 4 bases. In (b) the resulting fragment lengths are compared by electrophoresis.

variety of mechanisms more diverse than the sex life of *Homo sapiens*—is important because microbes have served both as invaluable tools for understanding gene transfer in nature, and also as the first subjects for artificial genetic modification.

In 1944 a 19-year-old medical student at Columbia University, Joshua Lederberg, began some experiments to determine how the DNA in Oswald Avery's experiments got into his smooth *pneumococci* to transform them. Two years later, working at Yale with the microbiologist Edward Tatum, he made the crucial breakthrough. He took two strains of bacteria, both requiring four different nutrients to grow. But one had the enzymes and thus the genes to make two of the nutrients, while the second strain was able to make the other two. When Lederberg put the bacteria together into a medium lacking all four nutrients, a new strain appeared that *was* able to grow. The chances of this resulting from random mutation were virtually zero. Lederberg and Tatum thus concluded that the four genes had come together by sexual **conjugation** between the two original strains.

We now know that 'male' or F+ bacteria possess a type of plasmid known as an F (fertility) factor, which determines the production of tiny hair-like pilli, through which DNA can be transferred by conjugation to 'female' (F−) bacteria lacking the F factor. One strand of the plasmid DNA is thought to pass over, carrying the genes in their normal linear order. Complementary strands are then synthesized in both the recipient and the donor. Both are then F+ cells. Sometimes F factors become integrated briefly with chromosomal DNA in a bacterium, and then take some of those genes with them during conjugation. Conjugation is thus one mechanism through which plasmids are spread through bacterial populations.

Another mechanism that transfers genes between bacteria is transduction, which was discovered by Joshua Lederberg and Norton Zinder. In this case, the DNA is ferried from the donor organism to the recipient inside a **bacteriophage**—a type of virus that attacks bacteria, rather than plants or animals. Like other viruses, phages consist of little more than nucleic acid wrapped in a protein coat. When a phage meets a susceptible bacterium, it becomes attached to the cell wall and injects its DNA into the cell. The phage DNA then redirects the cell's ribosomes, tRNAs, and other machinery to produce complete new phage particles, which are released twenty minutes or so later. Sometimes, however, fragments of bacterial DNA are incorporated in the new viruses and are in turn injected with the phage DNA into another bacterium.

Chasing the DNA

In 1952, Martha Chase and Alfred Hershey used a bacteriophage to provide another key piece of evidence that DNA, rather than protein, was the carrier of genetic information. They used two radioactive isotopes as 'labels' to determine whether DNA or protein entered the bacterial cell to initiate new phage production. One was an isotope of phosphorus (an element that occurs in DNA but not in the protein coat of phages) and the other an isotope of sulphur (which occurs in the protein but not in DNA).

Chase and Hershey first cultured phages in bacteria which, in turn, were growing in a medium containing chemicals labelled with the tell-tale radioactivity. This provided a stock of phages carrying both labels. Then they added the labelled phages to unlabelled bacteria, in order to see what happened to the labelled DNA and protein. The results indicated that the nucleic acid, but not the protein, entered the bacteria and triggered the synthesis of more phages.

Looking back on this work several years later, the pioneer virologist N. W. Pirie observed that while the conclusion proved to be correct, the figures for the analyses of protein and DNA that entered and remained outside the cell were less clear-cut than might have been expected. He suggested that the enthusiasm with which scientists accepted the result reflected their eagerness to prove that nucleic acids were indeed the carriers of genetic information.

Genes, mutations, and disease

In the next chapter, we shall turn from the advent and present
standing of molecular biology as a discipline of 'pure science',
to the emergence of applications in the form of techniques that
permit the conscious alteration of genetic material. In the
medical world, the prospect of modifying human genes sprang
originally from the recognition of the molecular basis of certain
diseases. One of the earliest examples was in 1949, when the
US chemist Linus Pauling traced sickle cell anaemia to a
specific defect in the structure of one molecule—haemoglobin.
Using electrophoresis, he demonstrated that haemoglobin from
sickle cell anaemia patients was distinct from normal haemoglobin. Adult haemoglobin is constructed of two alpha globin
chains, each 140 amino acids long, and two beta globin chains,
each with 146 amino acids. The sole abnormality in the
abnormal haemoglobins was the replacement of one amino
acid, glutamic acid, by valine at the sixth position in the beta
chain.

Sickle cell anaemia is an inherited disease. Other examples
of conditions attributable to an inherited mutation include
Huntington's disease, which causes progressive mental retardation and involuntary muscular movements, but does not
become manifest until about 35 years of age or even older. By
no means however are all genetic disorders familial. Some
disease-causing mutations or chromosomal abnormalities arise
during the formation of the gametes or the early development
of the fetus. One example is Down's syndrome, which causes
mental retardation, below-average stature, and other abnormalities. It usually arises from an error during meiosis, leading
to the child having 47 chromosomes instead of 46, with three
copies of chromosome 21 instead of the normal two copies. In
such cases the parents have the normal complement of
chromosomes. Similarly, normal genes are found in parents of
children with conditions caused by random mutations during
the formation of sperm or egg or during early development.

Most genetic disorders are maintained in the population by

both the passage of genes from parents to offspring and a steady input of new mutations. For reasons not yet entirely clear, certain conditions are linked particularly with errors in one sex or the other. Down's syndrome, for example, is associated more frequently with a mistake during meiosis on the mother's side than the father's. The reverse is true in retinoblastoma, a rare familial cancer of the retina.

Mutation can also give rise to cancer. If a mutation occurs in a DNA sequence known as a proto-oncogene, which normally codes for an enzyme or other protein essential to cell growth, it can push the normal process of mitosis out of control, leading to malignant growth.

Cells do have their own mechanisms for dealing with mutations. When, for example, two adjoining thymine bases become linked together (thus distorting the double helix and causing a mismatch during replication) a DNA repair enzyme splits the **dimer** bridge and restores normality. More complex excision-repair enzymes can snip out a damaged strand, assemble a new one to match the complementary strand, and stitch it in place.

Developmental genetics and cellular differentiation

Although everyone knows that the human gestation period is about nine months, it is less widely known that the basic body plan of the embryo is established very early, within the first four weeks of pregnancy when a woman is usually not even aware that she is pregnant. By the end of this period of active cell division the embryo is already recognizable as a miniature animal. It has a central nervous system, muscle, heart, and gut, together with extra-embryonic tissues that give rise to the placenta. In later development there is further **differentiation** of tissues and organs, and a great deal of growth sustained by nourishment from the mother's bloodstream. During this later phase the fetus becomes distinctly human, whereas earlier in development there is a striking similarity to other vertebrate embryos.

Early development, the establishment of the broad plan of the body, is a question of regional specification or how cells of different parts of the embryo become switched into appropriate pathways of development. Another aspect of early development is morphogenesis, which is how cellular and tissue movements give form to the embryo. Primitive streak formation is a process of very active morphogenesis which gives rise to an embryo with a clear head-to-tail axis. Subsequent migration of cells originally aligned along this axis is important in formation of the face and the peripheral nervous system, in the distribution of pigment cells in the skin, and in formation of muscles in the limbs.

We know that, with certain exceptions, all the nuclei of cells in the adult body contain a complete set of genes. So, for example, alpha and beta globin genes are present in kidney cell nuclei, even though these genes do not function in kidney cells because they are not transcribed into RNA. Cellular differentiation is fundamentally a question of controlling and co-ordinating patterns of gene activity so that genes are activated appropriately. Morphogenesis must ultimately depend upon gene activity but it also involves cellular properties that lie outside what is normally regarded as molecular biology.

From flies to man

Explanations of how embryos develop are relatively complex if even just the main aspects of morphogenesis, regional specification, and cellular differentiation are to be included. However, there has recently been great progress in the molecular genetical understanding of embryogenesis in one animal, the fruit fly *Drosophila*. Christine Nusslein-Volhard and her colleagues began this work by systematically identifying genes which control regional specification in the embryo. By combining genetics with molecular biology it has been possible to learn much of how the body plan of the larva develops from the egg. A picture is revealed in which there is first a maternal contribution involving a pattern of localized proteins or messenger RNAs, laid down in the egg. These localized molecules control patterns of gene activity in the nuclei of the embryo. They do this at a stage when many nuclei have formed in the embryo and these nuclei are distributed within a single cytoplasm—a feature of *Drosophila* development that does not occur in vertebrate development. Taking the head-to-tail axis of the embryo for consideration, the genes that are controlled by the maternal morphogens are the so-called gap genes. The gap genes in turn act in combination to set up the number and polarity of segments visible along the head-to-tail axis of the larva. They do this by controlling the segmentation genes. Many genes in this hierarchy have the role of activating particular homeotic selector genes in the correct place relative to the segmental pattern. The homeotic selector genes were in fact the first genes to be discovered, in the 1920s and 1930s, that affect regional specification in *Drosophila*. When mutated, these genes cause transformations of one part of the body into another, for example antennae into legs, and for this reason it was long ago realized that homeotic mutations must affect regional specification in a fundamental way.

Many of the genes in this developmental cascade, including the homeotic selector genes, encode transcription factors, whose function is to bind to DNA at control regions associated with particular genes and thereby to activate or repress their transcription. There are other genes in this cascade which act after cellularization of the embryo has taken place and which control specification by cell-to-cell interactions. These interactions involve signalling proteins which are actively secreted by one cell and which bind to receptor proteins on the surface of another cell.

As it is clear that homeotic selector genes encode transcription factors, it is presumed that they control the fate of the cells in which they are expressed by acting as 'master switches' which control batteries of other genes whose functioning determines the differentiation of the cell. These processes are yet to be elucidated.

In *Drosophila*, it is possible, at least in outline, to explain how a large number of genes interact to establish the segmental pattern of the larva. Conclusions that have been drawn from this work are that (i) impressively complete descriptions of regional specification can now be achieved, (ii) the number of interacting genes is large but not enormous, and (iii) it is evident that powerful genetics has been an essential tool in this field.

The small size, fragility, and development of mammalian embryos in the uterus have meant that progress in early mammalian embryology has been slow compared either with invertebrates such as *Drosophila* or the nematode worm, or with amphibian vertebrates which have been the subject of much classical embryology. But techniques for super-ovulation, for embryo culture and embryo modification, and most importantly techniques for isolating genes and for making transgenic animals, have revolutionized the field. Examples of these developments are discussed in later chapters. Perhaps the most remarkable contribution to the mammalian field has come from the *Drosophila* work. Genes that have been found to be crucial in fly development have been isolated and used as probes so that their mammalian counterparts can be isolated and studied. It has turned out that many of the fly genes do indeed have mammalian counterparts. A question then arises; do these mammalian genes have fundamental roles in the embryology of mammals, or is the resemblance to the fly genes simply due to a conservation of biochemical function with no role in regional specification in mammals? Answering this question is possible, using the new techniques of mammalian embryology. That the mammalian counterparts of the *Drosophila* homeotic genes *are* important in development seems to be evident from the finding that not only are the structures of the individual genes conserved, but indeed whole clusters of genes are conserved, with the orders of individual genes maintained within the clusters. Furthermore this order corresponds with the physical location of the expression pattern of the genes along the head-to-tail axis of the fly or mouse embryo. The reasons for this remarkable conservation are not known, but it hints at a conservation of function at a profound level.

Differentiated cells

The approach to developmental biology which has been described above could be called a 'forwards' approach. Genes are identified which are important in regional specification and their effects are followed through the developmental programme. As an alternative there is the 'backwards' approach. Here a terminally differentiated cell phenotype is examined for genes which control the genes whose activity is characteristic of the phenotype. Examples of characteristic genes are the globin genes in the red blood cell lineage and the antibody genes in lymphocytes. In such cases transcription factors have been identified whose function is to activate these characteristic genes in differentiating cells. One such example is the myoD transcription factor, which is involved in muscle cell differentiation. Importantly, it is found that expression of high amounts of myoD can actually cause certain non-muscle cells to differentiate into muscle. MyoD is a member of a large family of proteins which can interact directly with each other to form mixed dimers which have diverse properties in switching on and off different genes. Another member of the family is a gene involved in the causation of certain cancers, the proto-oncogene c-myc, which emphasizes the close relationship between normal cellular differentiation and its aberrant manifestation in cancer.

Intercellular signalling in development, differentiation, and homeostasis

Relating the activity of transcription factors, which are involved in complex networks of interacting proteins, to intercellular signalling molecules is crucial in understanding cellular differentiation. It has been discovered recently that the sites of activity (receptors) for the steroid hormones, vitamin D, and vitamin A are transcription factors whose activity is regulated by binding of the hormone or vitamin. Thus it is clear that the primary effects of these hormones and vitamins, which are active in differentiation and development, lie at the level of gene transcription. Discovering the roles of cellular receptors for other intercellular signalling molecules which are active in differentiation and development, such as growth factors, is a task in which progress has been made, particularly in respect of the pathways inside cells by which the initial perception of the signal by a receptor on the cell surface is transmitted to downstream functional effects within the cell. The depth of knowledge being gained is so profound that the current clinical applications, for example in developing new pharmaceuticals such as an anti-oestrogen for use in treatment of breast cancer, or vitamin A analogues in the treatment of certain leukaemias, are a small foretaste of what can be expected in coming decades.

Chapter Four

The Techniques of Molecular Biology

In 1965, the highly regarded medical journal the *Lancet* carried an article in which the Nobel prize-winning immunologist Sir Macfarlane Burnet insisted that there was no conceivable way in which what had been learned about protein synthesis and the genetic code could be applied for human benefit. However fascinating molecular biology might be as a scholarly achievement, Burnet argued, it had not produced anything of practical value, and was most unlikely to do so in future. Those comments already deserve to go into the archives alongside famed observations such as Lord Rutherford's alleged statement that no practical consequences could be expected from the splitting of the atom, or a former Astronomer Royal's statement that talk of space travel was 'bunk'. During the past twenty-five years, molecular biology has indeed begun to spawn applications, based on our new-found capacity to take a piece of DNA from one organism and join it artificially to one from another, to produce **recombinant DNA (rDNA)**. Genetic modification is the craft that harnesses this type of work.

In turn, genetic modification has fuelled the boom that has occurred over the last two decades in biotechnology—the exploitation of microbes and other types of cell to produce useful materials and facilitate industrial processes. Biotechnology itself is not new. In a sense it began with the ancient art of fermenting sugar to make alcoholic beverages, and led to the first mass production of antibiotics earlier this century. But these social and industrial activities were all dependent on living organisms as they existed in nature. The only scientific aids were techniques of identifying and selecting particularly effective strains. The advent of recombinant DNA has greatly extended the power, specificity, and range of biotechnology in its capacity to engineer novel organisms.

Excising and splicing DNA

The discoveries that led to the present possibilities for genetically modifying microbes and plants took place during the early 1970s. Herbert Boyer, working at the University of California Health Science Center in San Francisco, and Stanley Cohen at Stanford University found that it was possible to insert into bacteria genes they had removed from other bacteria (and subsequently from totally unrelated animal or plant cells). As described in more detail below, they first learned the trick of breaking down the DNA of a donor organism into manageable fragments. They achieved this by using **restriction endonucleases**, a type of bacterial enzyme discovered by Werner Arber, Hamilton Smith, and Daniel Nathans. Second, they discovered how to place such genes into a **vector**—often a bacteriophage or a plasmid. They could then employ the vector to ferry the selected fragment of DNA into the recipient bacterium. Once inside its new host, the transported gene divided as the cell divided, leading to a **clone** of cells each containing exact copies of the gene. This technique became known as gene cloning, and was followed by the selection of recipient cells containing the desired gene. Another type of genetic modification is the deletion of genes. A third is the direct modification of a gene to alter the protein it produces.

The enzymes used to cleave the DNA into pieces are highly specific in their action. Genes can therefore be removed and transferred from one organism to another with extraordinary precision. Such manœuvres contrast sharply with the much less predictable gene transfers that occur in nature or which arise from the breeding of animals for agricultural or show purposes. Moreover, they give us the capacity to splice together genes that would be unlikely to come together naturally. By mobilizing pieces of DNA in this way (including copies of human genes), genetic engineers are now fabricating genetically modified microbes for a wide range of applications in industry, medicine, and agriculture. Human insulin, identical to that made in the human pancreas, is one of the first commercial products to be produced by genetically modified bacteria. Such substances are manufactured by growing cultures of the modified microbe in nutrient medium inside a bioreactor (sometimes rather imprecisely called a fermenter).

Arising from the same discoveries that facilitated the new era of genetic modification are other exquisitely precise methods of studying and identifying segments of DNA. Sometimes loosely coupled together under the heading of recombinant DNA techniques, these depend upon the same enzymes that are used to snip out particular genes. Particularly widely used are DNA **probes**, short pieces of radioactively labelled DNA that stick very specifically to other, complementary pieces of DNA and thus provide a means of identifying them unambiguously.

The organism most often employed in these studies has been the bacterium *Escherichia coli*. Found in huge populations in the intestines of humans and other animals, *E. coli* is normally entirely innocuous (although certain strains, capable of producing toxins, can cause diarrhoea). The *E. coli* used in laboratory experiments has lost its ability to colonize the gut, as a result of being cultivated in artificial medium over many years. In some cases altered and foreign genes may be introduced not only into other bacteria, but also into yeasts, fungi, fruit flies, fertilized eggs, mammalian cells in culture, and some plants.

Switching genes on

Because certain genes regulate the production of proteins encoded by other gene sequences, it is not usually sufficient for only the DNA sequence responsible for a desired product (i.e. the structural gene) to be spliced into the DNA of another organism. The gene must be expressed—that is, it must be 'switched on' by the associated regulatory elements in the DNA. Biotechnologists thus exploit both structural and controlling genes. They transfer the former (to give organisms the capacity to make new products) along with the latter (which turn on their corresponding structural genes, often to boost the synthesis of proteins far beyond their natural level).

In industry, the designers of manufacturing plants often arrange that a substance is made in response to an appropriate signal—typically the presence of a particular nutrient in the culture medium. One approach makes use of the lactose operon. This is the stretch of DNA that codes for the enzymes which certain bacteria use to digest lactose and also for the operator which, in the presence of this sugar, switches on these genes. The lactose operon can be spliced into a plasmid with foreign DNA immediately alongside. Exposed to lactose, a bacterium carrying such a plasmid begins to make not only the enzymes required to use the sugar but also the protein encoded by the foreign DNA.

Cleaving DNA

While the basic idea of transferring genes between cells is quickly explained, the actual practice is more complicated. The scale of the problem can be gauged from the astronomical numbers involved. The genome of E. coli, for example, contains 4,800,000 pairs of bases, while the human genome consists of three thousand million (i.e. one billion) base pairs. Even a single human chromosome carries many millions of base pairs. How, therefore, can one locate a particular gene and detach it from the rest in order to transplant it elsewhere? The answer is that it is virtually impossible to do this in one or two simple steps, as one might excise a piece of text in an article and move it elsewhere, either on paper or on a word processor screen. DNA carries a vast quantity of information, and its meaning cannot be scanned as easily as one can peruse the pages of a book. A more ingenious strategy has had to be developed.

The first step in this strategy is to snip up the DNA into smaller pieces, each containing one or just a few genes. This is achieved using restriction endonucleases; the enzymes that cut DNA in very precise ways. They do so by recognizing particular stretches of bases (usually four to six pairs, termed recognition sequences) and then snipping each strand of the double helix at a particular place (see Fig. 4.1). Whenever the recognition sequence appears in the long DNA chain, an endonuclease makes a cut. And whenever the same enzymes are used to break up a certain piece of DNA, they always produce the same set of fragments. The cuts occur in such a way as to produce pieces of double helix with short stretches of single-stranded DNA at each end. These are known as sticky ends. As in the natural process of DNA replication, bases have an inherent propensity (under the right chemical conditions) to join up with their partners—A with T, and G with C. So too with sticky ends. For example, the sequence T–T–A–A– will tend to reassociate with –A–A–T–T. Genetic scientists use another type of enzyme, **DNA ligase**, to make the union permanent.

This is the key principle of gene splicing—the use of two types of enzyme to cut out one piece of DNA and then to attach it to another piece. Several hundred different restriction endonucleases have now been identified and incorporated in the genetic scientist's toolkit. Each is a precision instrument for fragmenting DNA in a particular way. Some recognize different base sequences; others recognize the same sequence but snip at a different point within or next to the sequence.

Once a piece of DNA has been broken up into a mixture of different fragments, these can be separated by electrophoresis in a jelly-like material called an agarose gel. Larger fragments move more slowly than smaller ones down the running track. The result is a pattern, with the smallest pieces furthest from

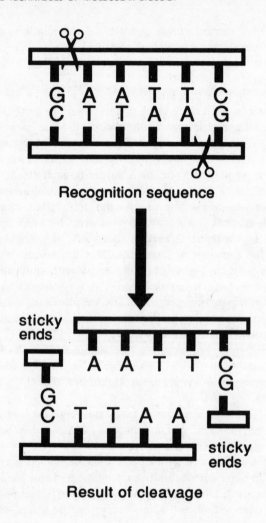

Recognition sequence

sticky
ends

sticky
ends

Result of cleavage

Fig. 4.1 Cleaving DNA using a restriction endonuclease

the starting-point. DNA fragments of one particular length can also be taken from the gel and exposed to another restriction enzyme, yielding even smaller pieces.

Ferrying the gene into a bacterium

The next stage is the insertion of foreign DNA into a vector, which is usually either a plasmid or a bacteriophage. Vectors are used to ferry desirable genes into the organism that is to be engineered. Plasmids first attracted attention as possible vectors because these self-replicating circular pieces of DNA can become incorporated in the bacterial nucleus and then later detach from it, carrying genes with them. Plasmids seem to have evolved as a natural mechanism for moving genes around among bacteria. Likewise with bacteriophages. As well as invading bacterial cells and immediately triggering the manufacture of new phage particles, they too can become integrated into the bacterial chromosome and carry genes away when they break free some time later (a process that can be stimulated artificially).

To insert foreign DNA into a vector, the genetic scientist first splits open the plasmid or phage by adding the same endonuclease that is used to split the DNA of the donor organism into short fragments (see Fig. 4.2). This creates sticky ends complementary to those on the fragments of foreign DNA to be transplanted. A fragment thus fits neatly into the gap in the vector DNA, where it is firmly annealed by DNA ligase. The aim is thus to incorporate a foreign gene and its regulatory sequences into the vector. (In this random process, some of the sticky ends of the vector may, of course, simply find each other and rejoin to reconstitute the original. Also, DNA fragments which do not contain the particular foreign gene will be incorporated.) Next, the plasmid or phage is allowed to infect a bacterium (often *E. coli*) in which it can replicate. Phage infection is highly efficient, but the alternative approach, transformation by plasmids passing through the cell surface, may have to be facilitated by chemical treatment. Once inside,

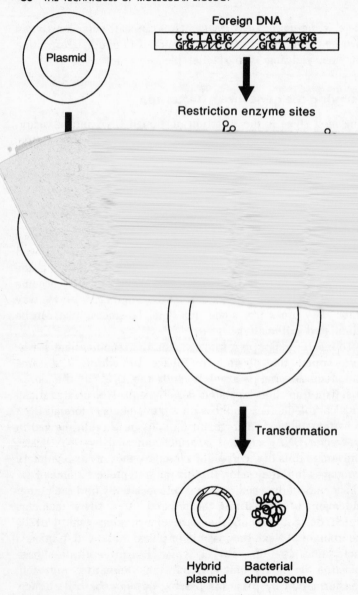

Fig. 4.2 Ferrying foreign DNA into a bacterium

method of gene copying, which has revolutionized several aspects of molecular biology since it was introduced only a few years ago, is the **polymerase chain reaction (PCR)**. Devised originally by researchers at the Cetus Corporation in California, the PCR is a method of copying DNA chemically in a test-tube in just a few hours. Although it does not use living cells, the process can make DNA grow exponentially because it takes place in successive steps, each doubling the amount of DNA.

The key to the technique is that one must know the sequences of short stretches of DNA on either side of the gene to be copied. A gene machine is used to make two primers— single strands of DNA, one complementary to one of the flanking sequences and the other to the other. The DNA double helix containing the gene is then untwisted and separated. When the two primers are added, each binds to its complementary flanking sequence. Next, the enzyme DNA polymerase is added. It immediately extends not only the primers, but also the target gene too. This series of three steps, each requiring a different temperature, comprises one cycle of the PCR. With an appropriate succession of temperature changes, as few as twenty cycles can generate approximately a million times the amount of the original target sequence (see Fig. 4.4).

There are many emerging applications of the PCR outside the realm of genetics. For example, US scientists used it in 1990 to investigate Lyme disease, an infection that was first recognized as a distinct disease in the mid-1970s. Lyme disease is carried by ticks, which pass on the infective agent, a spirochaete called *Borrelia burgdorferi*, to humans. By examining specimens from ticks in various museum collections, the researchers were able to demonstrate that DNA characteristic of the spirochaete—and presumably therefore the parasite itself—had existed as early as the 1940s, long before the infection was formally recognized. Applied to stored tissue taken from patients earlier this century, the PCR has also been employed to establish that the AIDS virus existed several decades before its apparent emergence for the first time in the USA in the early 1980s.

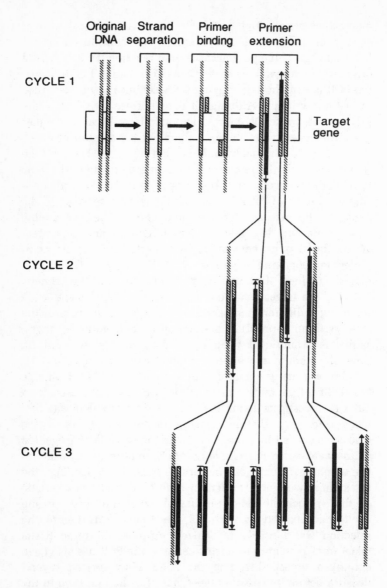

Fig. 4.4 Polymerase chain reaction for making multiple copies of a gene

Modification with proteins

Genetic modification as discussed earlier in this chapter involves the transfer of genes from one organism to another. A more elementary manœuvre is the simple deletion of a gene coding for an unwanted protein. A third variation on this theme is the direct modification of a gene, to make a correspondingly altered protein. This is called protein engineering. One application is to alter the amino acid sequence of enzymes, so as to produce molecules less sensitive to heat or having greater catalytic power. This can be achieved by site directed mutagenesis—a method of altering a gene at a very specific point.

The first step in this process is to separate the two DNA strands. A gene machine is then used to make a sequence of bases complementary to that of a strand coding for the part of the protein that is to be altered. The match is perfect except for a single error—perhaps a G replaces a T that would normally pair with A. As most of the bases are complementary, the two strands bind together. The remainder of the gene sequence (which is, of course, normal in structure) is then built up in the usual way, on the basis of the coded information in the other strand. The next step is to insert the entire piece of double-stranded DNA into a bacterium. When the organism begins to grow, it assembles a double-stranded gene from each of its strands. When the bacterium divides, one of the daughter cells receives a gene copied from the normal strand. The other receives a gene copied from the abnormal gene. It therefore produces a 'mutant' protein, altered in accordance with the instructions in the fragment made with the gene machine.

Site directed mutagenesis has been used to correct—in the test-tube—the defect in the gene that is responsible for thalassaemia. This is a blood disease caused by a single mutation in the globin gene. In place of a codon for an amino acid is a 'stop' codon. The protein-synthesizing machinery thus delivers a truncated form of globin, which fails to perfom its normal role of carrying oxygen around the body. When the correct codon is inserted, the mutated gene produces normal globin.

To arrange changes in a protein more extensive than a single amino acid, protein engineers use the technique of cassette mutagenesis. In this case a DNA segment of twenty to thirty bases is snipped out and replaced by the desired sequence made in a gene machine.

The techniques for modifying proteins are now being applied to antibodies, the protective proteins which are manufactured by the body in response to the antigenic stimuli of invading micro-organisms. These applications, which are based on the production of large quantities of monoclonal antibodies of high purity, will be discussed in Chapter 7.

Chapter Five

Modifying Micro-organisms

Microbes as workhorses

By definition, microbes can be seen only under a microscope. Yet they are both ubiquitous and essential to life as we know it. From the cradle to the grave, we are surrounded by astronomical numbers of them. There are some 100,000 microbes on every square centimetre of skin, while a teaspoonful of soil contains at least two billion. The microbial world also includes vast numbers of different species and strains. Although some microbes are agents of disease, the majority are beneficial, breaking down dead tissues, recycling elements, and helping plants to assimilate nitrogen from the air. Because microbes can reproduce much more quickly than higher organisms, they have a correspondingly rapid rate of evolution, spawning variants to exploit changes in the environment that are favourable to their survival. Several different mechanisms are responsible for a rich pattern of horizontal gene flow through the microbial world.

By making cheese, bread, and alcoholic beverages, we have been exploiting microbes from time immemorial. Earlier this century, scientists began to harness microbes more deliberately to make specific substances. During World War I, the émigré German chemist Chaim Weizmann, then in Manchester, developed a process in which the bacterium *Clostridium acetobutylicum* produced acetone, a solvent required in the manufacture of explosives. Then, during World War II, another émigré German chemist, Ernst Chain, and the Australian pathologist Howard Florey, working in Oxford, launched the antibiotic revolution by purifying penicillin from the mould *Penicillium notatum*.

In the beginning, such processes were based on growing naturally occurring microbes. Gradually, however, researchers improved on nature. First, they learned to alter conditions (for example, by adding certain nutrients) so that the organisms synthesized more of the desired products. Secondly, they devised methods of screening large numbers of strains very quickly to locate high-yielding microbes. Thirdly, they irradiated microbes, to increase the mutation rate and thus the chances of finding particularly effective strains.

Penicillin—the first antibiotic

The development of penicillin, although it occurred long before it became possible to modify genes, was one of the outstanding developments in the use of microbes to produce life-saving drugs. In 1928, at St Mary's Hospital in London, Alexander Fleming noticed that a mould had contaminated a culture of *staphylococci* (bacteria that cause skin and other infections). Later identified as *Penicillium notatum*, the mould seemed to have produced something that had attacked the bacteria. Fleming named the unidentified substance penicillin, but the chemists he approached were unable to purify the material. Fleming thought that it might be used simply as a laboratory tool, to inhibit the growth of sensitive bacteria in cultures of other, insensitive strains.

The idea of administering penicillin to treat infections was taken up vigorously by Howard Florey, Ernst Chain, and others at the Sir William Dunn School of Pathology, Oxford, nearly a decade later. The imminent need to treat large numbers of infected war wounds provided one motive for this work. In a project led by Florey, Chain, together with Norman Heatley, succeeded in extracting and purifying penicillin. Shown to be dramatically effective in curing certain bacterial infections, first in laboratory animals and then in humans, penicillin was immediately heralded as a wonder drug. It became the first of the modern generation of antibiotics, transforming medical practice, and leading another decade later to the so-called new penicillins made by chemically modifying the penicillin molecule to make it more effective in various ways.

In 1941, because demand for penicillin far exceeded the output of the Oxford laboratory and because industry was being disrupted by enemy bombing, Florey and Heatley visited the USA and secured help in organizing mass production of the antibiotic. Before leaving Britain, they smeared the linings of their coats with *Penicillium* spores, which could be recovered later if the cultures in Oxford were lost following a German invasion.

Making pharmaceuticals by genetic modification

DNA modification is the latest innovation in fabricating pedigree organisms, particularly for the pharmaceutical industry. By far the largest number of current applications of genetic modification are in the fields of human and animal health care. The hormone insulin for the treatment of diabetics, for example, was for decades extracted laboriously from the pancreas of cows and pigs. Now it is being manufactured by growing huge cultures of bacteria into which a human insulin gene has been inserted. Diabetes, which affects 6 per cent of individuals, takes two forms. Juvenile onset diabetes is caused by destruction of the cells that produce the hormone. Maturity onset diabetes is associated with obesity and a relative deficiency of insulin. Recombinant insulin has now become the treatment of choice for juvenile diabetes.

Human growth hormone, produced by bacteria carrying the relevant gene, is used to treat children with pituitary dwarfism, who would otherwise become adults of abnormally short stature. Freedom from virus contamination is a major advantage of this method of production as compared with extraction from animal tissues. The dangers are illustrated by an incident that occurred in the late 1980s. Three individuals, who in the

1960s and 1970s had received human growth hormone extracted from the pituitary glands of human cadavers, died from Creutzfeldt-Jacob disease, caused by contamination of the hormone preparation. This led to the withdrawal of hormone prepared in that way, and accelerated the development of genetically manufactured hormone made in *E. coli*.

Interferon, over-publicized in the past as an alleged cure-all for cancer, is now known to consist of several different varieties. Several of these have been produced by recombinant DNA methods and have emerged as promising treatments against some cancers and some virus infections. Interferon-alpha is firmly established as an effective treatment for hairy cell leukaemia, while genital warts and other benign tumours associated with human papillomavirus infection also respond well to interferon-alpha. Genetically manufactured interferons are also proving effective against hepatitis B, and against hepatitis C if given at the correct time.

Colony stimulating factors, which boost the production of white blood cells and play major roles in the immune response against infection, are also being made by genetically altered organisms. One of these, granulocyte colony stimulating factor, is useful as a means of overcoming a hazardous side-effect of many anti-cancer drugs which is their propensity to impair the production of white blood cells and thus leave the patient vulnerable to infection. Granulocyte-macrophage colony stimulating factor has been given to AIDS patients to boost the formation of white cells. Interleukin-2, which regulates the growth and differentiation of white cells, is also beginning to show promise against cancer, as is tumour necrosis factor.

Erythropoietin is a growth factor, produced in the kidneys, that stimulates the manufacture of red blood cells in the bone marrow. Although it can be made by bacteria carrying copies of the relevant human gene, the preferred workhorse is a line of cells derived from Chinese hamsters. The reason for this is that, in hamster cells, the gene product is modified further after translation making the final product closer to the human version than that made in bacteria. Erythropoietin is already proving invaluable in combating the anaemia suffered by people with chronic kidney failure who are being treated by dialysis and otherwise need repeated blood transfusions. It has also been illicitly used by athletes in efforts to increase their stock of red blood cells and thus their sporting performance.

One of the most recent innovations in genetic modification is the production of human luteinizing hormone (the agent that brings about ovulation) by mammalian cells carrying copies of the relevant human genes. This represents a major advance on conventional extraction of the hormone from human urine, for use in the treatment of infertility and in *in vitro* fertilization programmes. As well as coming from a more dependable source of supply, the manufactured hormone is more easily standardized so that the correct dosage can be given.

Another innovation is the use of tissue plasminogen activator (tPA) following coronary thrombosis. tPA occurs naturally in very small quantities in the bloodstream, where it prevents unwanted clots from forming. Injected quickly into heart attack victims, the genetically modified version is effective in breaking down blood clots that block the blood vessels. Blood clotting proteins, which are deficient in patients with haemophilia, can also be made by genetically altered bacteria.

Some types of emphysema and associated diseases are accompanied by inadequate levels of particular proteins in the bloodstream. These normally guard lung tissue from attack by powerful digestive enzymes released accidentally from scavenging white blood cells. The major protective protein, alpha-1-antitrypsin, is being produced by bacteria carrying recombinant DNA. There are high hopes that it will prove to be valuable in the treatment of emphysema in heavy smokers and other diseases such as respiratory distress syndrome in infants.

Atriopeptin is a hormone produced not in a gland but inside the heart. In fact, several atriopeptins have now been characterized, and shown to play different roles in controlling blood pressure. Produced by genetic modification, they are expected to prove of value in medicine.

An emerging application of molecular biology is the development of hybrid antibiotics. These are made by altering the genes responsible for antibiotic production in fungi and bacteria, so that they make antibiotics with correspondingly altered molecules. Hybrid antibiotics could help to circumvent the problems posed by bacteria that are resistant to conventional antibiotics. Site directed mutagenesis has also been employed to alter the structure of hormones, offering the prospect of hybrid hormones with more selective actions than their natural counterparts.

A new generation of vaccines

Many of the vaccines used for immunization are based on principles that have changed little over the past century. Some, such as Salk poliomyelitis vaccine, consist of microbes that are killed but retain their ability to induce immunity. Others, including Sabin polio vaccine, consist of a live virus which has been weakened so as to prevent it causing disease (attenuated) and which can pass from the vaccinated person to other individuals in the community thereby making them immune to polio as well. Either way, traditional vaccines require the cultivation of large quantities of the microbe. In some cases (leprosy, for example), this is very difficult.

Genetic modification offers two prospects. First, vaccine makers can grow harmless bacteria into which they have inserted genes coding for the proteins (antigens) that trigger the production of protective antibodies against disease-causing microbes. The proteins can then be purified using monoclonal antibodies. Vaccines against hepatitis B, tetanus, and diphtheria, and foot-and-mouth disease in cattle have been made in this way. The second approach is to fabricate live vaccines. This too can be done by inserting genes into a microbe that is itself harmless but which serves as a carrier for the relevant genes and thus produces antibody-inducing antigens. Because this involves the deliberate release of a genetically altered organism, we shall now consider this area more closely.

From containment to release

Microbes used to make pharmaceuticals are confined inside culture vessels, and killed once they have done their work. Moreover, even if they were to escape accidentally, bacteria modified to over-produce proteins such as insulin are thought to be extremely ill-fitted to establish themselves in the outside world. Now, however, there are plans to release genetically modified microbes deliberately into the environment, for practical benefits in medicine, agriculture, and other fields. We shall consider four out of many potential applications of this sort.

One-shot vaccines

Salmonella typhimurium, a bacterium commonly responsible for food poisoning, is now being used as the basis of a novel type of vaccine. Geneticists have removed the genes coding for certain enzymes, thereby disabling the bacterium and ensuring that it lives only long enough to provoke immunity but does not invade the body or cause disease. Although the organism arrives at its customary habitat in the intestine, it dies out after a few days. But genes can also be added, giving the bacterium the capacity to make antigens that trigger antibody production against many other infections, including tetanus, influenza, and even malaria. More than one foreign gene can be inserted into the same bacterium, one shot of which could confer immunity against several different diseases.

Another possible carrier for other antigens is vaccinia virus, which was used for immunization against smallpox until the disease was rendered extinct in 1978. Genes taken from influenza, hepatitis B, rabies, rinderpest, and other viruses have been transferred into vaccinia. A modified vaccinia carrying genes from the rabies virus has been tested in the wild in Europe in recent years and found to be effective in inducing immunity to rabies in foxes.

Some researchers have urged caution in the use of vaccinia

in humans. They point out that occasional side-effects, tolerable when vaccinia was deployed against the killer disease smallpox, are not acceptable when the target disease is much less threatening. Other critics have warned that there could be complications if vaccinia vaccines were used in a continent such as Africa where many people have been infected by the human immunodeficiency virus (HIV), which impairs the body's immune response to infection.

Viruses against forest pests

A second type of genetic modification is centred on naturally occurring baculoviruses, which attack certain insects but do not infect plants or other animals. Although some non-modified baculoviruses are already available commercially as living insecticides, they tend to act too slowly, allowing time for pests to continue damaging their host plants for days or even weeks. The specificity of baculoviruses, combined with the disadvantage of residues left by chemical insecticides, has encouraged scientists at the Institute of Virology and Environmental Microbiology in Oxford to set out to make them more effective than their natural counterparts.

One possibility is to incorporate bacterial genes coding for toxins, creating viruses with heightened killing power. Preliminary work has shown that a released baculovirus can be traced through a base sequence placed as a label into a non-coding region of its genome. Field studies have also been conducted with a virus genetically crippled by deleting the gene coding for its protein coat. The results indicated not only that the 'naked' virus had retained its ability to cause disease, but also that it could not persist in the environment—thus limiting its possible spread or interaction with other baculoviruses. One intended target for this work is the pine beauty moth, a pest responsible for considerable damage to pine plantations in Scotland.

A bacterium that prevents frost damage

Scientists at the University of California, Berkeley, and Advanced Genetic Sciences of Oakwood, California, have devised a novel strategy to combat frost damage to crops, which causes losses of over one billion dollars every year in the USA. They began by investigating why plant tissues do not always freeze, even when chilled well below the point at which they would be expected to do so. The explanation hinges on bacteria which act as 'nucleation centres' for the formation of ice crystals on leaf surfaces thereby causing frost damage. In the absence of these bacteria, plants can survive otherwise damagingly low temperatures. The researchers decided to identify the genes in the bacteria responsible for ice nucleation, delete them, and spray the altered bacteria onto plants. They hoped that the altered organism would compete with and replace the natural varieties, or prevent them from colonizing the plants in the first place. The Californian team achieved this with a strain of *Pseudomonas syringae*. The 'ice minus' bacteria reduced frost injury to strawberries by 20–90 per cent (as compared with untreated plants) in greenhouse experiments. When tested in the open air, it provided a practically useful degree of frost protection, and did not become widely disseminated or cause any hazards.

Bacteria to deliver pesticides

A fourth candidate for controlled release is a novel type of pesticide developed at Monsanto Agricultural Products. The starting-point was *Bacillus thuringiensis*, a bacterium that parasitizes the leaf-munching larvae of the gypsy moth and other caterpillars that attack important agricultural crops. Farmers have been using commercial preparations of this organism for a quarter of a century to protect plants such as cabbage, cotton, beans, and potatoes. To ensure continued protection, however, crops must be sprayed not just once but repeatedly. The Monsanto scientists decided to circumvent this problem by cloning the gene responsible for the toxicity of *B. thuringiensis* and transferring it to *Pseudomonas fluorescens*, a harmless bacterium that colonizes plant roots. Applied to seeds or soil at the time of planting, the engineered organism could thus afford long-term protection against soil-borne pests.

Medicines from viruses

Although viruses consist of little more than nucleic acid wrapped in a protein coat, and can reproduce themselves only by invading living cells, they might be used in future to make pharmaceutical products. Particularly promising candidates are the baculoviruses, which occur in nature as parasites of the cotton bollworm, pine beauty moth, and other pests. When a caterpillar eats a piece of leaf contaminated with baculovirus, the virus begins to attack virtually every cell in its body, commanding them to make the virus protein called polyhedrin and killing the insect in a few days. Geneticists have now learned to delete the gene coding for polyhedrin and replace it with any one of a large number of foreign genes. Already, the genes for more than thirty human proteins have been incorporated into baculoviruses, which could be used to make hepatitis-B vaccine and other pharmaceuticals. Proponents of this system argue that it is likely to be much cheaper than growing genetically modified bacteria in bulk cultures. An insectary of a few thousand caterpillars could produce several grams of human protein. This could mean vaccine proteins at a tenth of their present cost.

A genetically modified foodstuff

In 1990, the UK became the first country to sanction the development of a food product containing a live, genetically modified organism. Approval was given to the use of a strain of the baker's yeast, *Saccharomyces cerevisiae*, developed by the Dutch company Gist-Brocades. The organism was produced by inserting a novel DNA sequence into its genome. The sequence consisted of two of the yeast's own genes, which code for maltase and maltose permease and thus govern the capacity to use maltose (malt sugar), together with new promoter genes taken from another strain of the same species. The aim was to produce a yeast that would take up and digest maltose more efficiently and thereby produce carbon dioxide, which makes bread rise, more quickly than before.

Is gene splicing inherently safe?

During the early debate over gene splicing, some researchers called for a moratorium on further work because they suspected that such artificial gene transfers were categorically different from those that occurred in nature. Today, most scientists find it virtually impossible to draw any such hard-and-fast dividing line. This is because natural gene flow has turned out to be far richer and more diverse than was thought hitherto.

At least some recombinant DNA modifications yield organisms that cannot be distinguished from those that have acquired their new genes in nature. A penicillin resistance gene, for example, can be inserted into a bacterium sensitive to penicillin. But this has been happening for many years in the field. Exposed to antimicrobial drugs widely used in human and veterinary medicine, bacteria containing plasmids with resistance genes have proliferated at the expense of those lacking them. Plasmids carrying resistance have also been transferred from one bacterium to another. Although resistance genes are inserted differently when spliced artificially, it is impossible to distinguish such an organism by its behaviour from one that acquires its drug-resistance naturally.

Scientists' new-found ability to insert chosen genes with exquisite precision also makes it possible to determine with greater accuracy how a recipient micro-organism will behave afterwards. Clearly, some possible insertions would be foolhardy—introducing a cancer gene into a bacterium capable of colonizing human intestines, for example. Such transfers could not occur accidentally and would not be carried out consciously except, perhaps, in biological warfare research, which because of its classified nature is beyond the scope of this book.

Safety and deliberate release

Microbes to be released into the environment are not only invisible to the naked eye, they are also alive, and will be exposed to other living creatures and to the natural elements too. So they could not be recalled in their entirety should anything go wrong. How, then, can we assess possible dangers in releasing microbes into the environment?

First, we can forecast a good deal about the behaviour of a microbe by studying its biology. A bacterium dependent upon a particular nutrient, for example, is certain to die out in an environment lacking that substance. Knowledge of a microbe's nutritional needs and of the temperatures at which it grows will permit predictions to be made about those habitats in which it will prosper.

One particular need is to ensure that a released microbe is not fitted, by its biological characteristics, to behave as an opportunistic pathogen—an organism that does not normally cause disease but can do so under certain circumstances. Although it has certainly not been released deliberately, *Legionella pneumophila* is a good example of an opportunistic pathogen. This bacterium occurs commonly, and without apparent harm to humans, in many natural water systems. But if it proliferates inside cooling towers and is then disseminated as a fine mist, the same organism can cause the potentially fatal Legionnaires' disease.

Another way to prevent possible dangers arising from the release of a genetically modified microbe is to to make it incapable of long-term survival. That is the strategy behind the new *Salmonella* vaccines now being developed. Such an approach would, of course, be totally inappropriate for a microbe such as a vaccine virus whose *raison d'être* was, like Sabin polio vaccine, wider dissemination in the community.

Indeed, present-day polio vaccines illustrate a crucial point about the release of a living organism into the environment. Sabin vaccine consists of a weakened though living virus, which is taken (often on a sugar lump) by mouth. One advantage of this type of immunization is that the virus is shed in the faeces of inoculated infants. It can thus be passed on to others, who become infected and therefore immune even without being vaccinated themselves. The corresponding disadvantage is the occurrence of extremely rare changes in the Sabin virus, making it capable of causing paralytic polio. Such reversion cannot take place with the Salk polio vaccine, which consists of non-living virus. This has to be administered by injection, and does not, of course, provoke immunity in people who have not received the vaccine.

The dilemma of choosing between a live and killed vaccine, which will be even sharper for genetically manufactured vaccines, is illustrated by experience in the Netherlands. When polio vaccines first became available, the Dutch government, unusually among European countries, decided to adopt the Salk rather than the Sabin version for its routine immunization programme. Since then, although polio has become virtually extinct as in other countries practising mass vaccination, there have been occasional outbreaks of the paralytic disease in an extreme Protestant sect whose members decline immunization on principle. Yet the children affected by these outbreaks might have escaped the disease had Holland chosen the Sabin virus, which would have circulated in the community and induced immunity even among unvaccinated individuals.

Lessons from previous experience

We can also learn from the past. Humans have for many years been releasing astronomical populations of (non-genetically modified) microbes into the environment. Sewage treatment plants are by no means totally isolated from the environment, and considerable quantities of sewage sludge are dumped onto agricultural land in many countries. Yet aside from those occasions when treatment plants break down, and those places where the technology has not been fully adopted, this massive off-loading of micro-organisms into our environment seems to occur without harm. Likewise, we have vast experience of both human and veterinary vaccines that have been genetically altered (though not, until very recently, by recombinant DNA techniques).

Man has long introduced foreign species into new environments. Over 100 different pests have been effectively controlled by introducing and establishing a species that is a natural enemy of the nuisance species. In particular, microbes such as *B. thuringiensis* have been cultivated and consciously released, without known hazard, to combat other forms of life which are inimical to crops. Although this bacterium possesses the machinery for transferring its toxin gene, no adverse environmental effects have been noted during more than twenty years of world-wide use.

We have particular experience of releasing *Rhizobium*, a bacterium that forms nodules on the roots of leguminous plants such as peas, clover, and alfalfa. In this symbiotic association, the rhizobia provide the plant with nitrogen 'fixed' in an assimilable form from the atmosphere. Around the beginning of this century, microbiologists realized that they could encourage nodulation, and thus boost the supply of nitrogen to plants, by inoculating seeds with these naturally occurring organisms. Ever since then, an industry has existed to supply preparations to farmers. Millions of hectares of land are now treated with rhizobia every year, without any adverse repercussions on health or the environment.

An ecological perspective

One lesson from the use of rhizobia is that an organism introduced into a new environment will persist only if it finds a suitable niche—a set of favourable environmental conditions to which it is peculiarly well adapted. This points to another source of insight—ecology—in predicting likely consequences when a genetically altered organism arrives in a new environment. Making an ecological analysis means taking the broadest possible perspective on how a new microbe or plant will interact not only with its target organism (such as a plant inoculated with pesticidal bacteria) but with other living things too. Ecology, which focuses on entire communities of plants, animals, and microbes and their complex interactions, can provide the most comprehensive guidance about likely changes following the introduction of a new species.

Monitoring microbes after release

For the foreseeable future at least, it will be important to determine how organisms behave after they are disseminated in the environment. Does a bacterium introduced into a wheat field disappear quickly, because it is unable to compete with the natural flora? Or does it proliferate and become established in the area where it was released? How far if at all is the organism transported away from the initial site? Answers to such questions are important in building a knowledge base against which to assess the behaviour of other organisms in future.

Methods are already well established for enumerating microbes in the environment. They are accurate and reliable, but have lower limits of detection—about ten organisms per gram in the case of soil. They also provide total counts, or counts of particular groups such as bacteria of intestinal origin, whose numbers are taken as a guide to the safety of water supplies. More discriminating approaches are used to detect particular species, especially when present in exceedingly small numbers. The investigator takes a sample of the material (such as food, soil, or a swab from a patient's throat) and inoculates it into nutrient medium especially favourable to growth of the organism in question, and/or places it in a selective medium that discourages the growth of others.

Even more specific is the use of fluorescence microscopy to reveal an individual strain of bacterium or virus. This depends upon the lock-and-key interaction between an antibody and its corresponding antigen which (through an associated fluorescent dye) betrays the presence of the microbe carrying it. Most discriminating of all are labelled DNA probes to identify particular DNA sequences. In contrast to culturing techniques, which indicate simply the existence and numbers of particular organisms, DNA probes pinpoint specific genes.

One problem is posed by bacteria that are alive but do not show up through conventional screening techniques. Studies on *Vibrio cholerae* (the agent of cholera) and *Legionella pneumophila*, for example, indicate that a proportion of cells may be viable yet incapable of growing when screened using nutrient medium. Fluorescence microscopy or gene probes are necessary to reveal bacteria in this condition.

Monitoring introduced genes

Marker genes, as incorporated in baculoviruses, can be used to trace both organisms and genes. Monsanto scientists have taken genes from *E. coli* and introduced them as markers into *P. aureofaciens*, which they hope to exploit in delivering pesticides to plant roots as they have done with *P. fluorescens*. The genes give the bacterium the capacity to utilize lactose, which can be exploited to indicate the organism's presence when inoculated onto a culture plate. The tracking system has proved effective in detecting a single bacterium within a background of one thousand million other bacterial cells.

It is also important to assess whether a plasmid carrying a spliced gene is likely to travel further and enter other, unrelated microbes. Under a European Community risk assessment programme, British, German, and French scientists have released *Rhizobium* bacteria containing a marker gene coding for resistance to certain antibiotics, as a label to determine to what extent genes are transferred to other rhizobia already in the soil. Methods of identifying plasmids have been employed for several years for purposes such as following the spread of drug-resistance around the world, and will be of value in assessing the frequency with which released microbes exchange plasmids with the existing flora.

Surveillance of this sort cannot hope to be comprehensive, in the sense of providing machinery capable of detecting every single gene movement. Horizontal gene flow in the microbial world is so rich that this would be an unrealistic goal. Current tests with marker genes will, however, indicate the likelihood of plasmids and the genes they carry being ferried else-where—and the possible consequences. One alternative strategy for dealing with this problem is, of course, for organisms to be altered so that there is a very low possibility that an introduced gene will travel beyond its original carrier.

Chapter Six

Modifying Plants and Crops

Breeding better plants

Our earliest and most important feat of plant breeding seems to have been the fabrication of maize, some 10,000 years ago. Maize is quite different from its nearest wild relatives, teosinte and tripsacum. These are grasses that produce seed in a tassel at the top of the plant, whereas maize produces its seed on bulky ears growing out of the stalk halfway up. Because it appeared in an evolutionary instant, maize is almost certainly a product of human intervention, based initially on the simple selection of seed for propagation and the intercrossing of odd-looking plants, before more sophisticated breeding techniques were applied. Maize cannot grow as a weed, and does not occur in the wild, because the kernels are so firmly attached to the ears that they do not fall off. Having no natural dispersal mechanism, it is entirely dependent on human beings for its survival. Even if an ear is left in a field and becomes buried in the soil, the plants are so crowded together when the kernels germinate that they do not generally flower.

Over the centuries and particularly during the decades of the past century, plant breeding has become an increasingly precise art. Crosses between existing varieties, complemented to some degree by the techniques of mutation and selection like those used for microbes, have produced higher yielding varieties of maize, wheat, rice, and other crops. Together with improvements in fertilizers, pesticides, herbicides, and irrigation techniques, these developments have played a major part in meeting the world's growing need for food. To take one of many comparable statistics, the average yield of maize per hectare in the USA more than tripled between 1930 and 1975. Advances of this sort were reflected during the Green Revolution that helped to boost food production in the Third World during the 1950s and 60s.

Although twentieth-century plant breeding has been a considerable advance on the crude hybridization and selection procedures of earlier centuries, several problems remain. One is that while breeders would like to introduce specific genes of agronomic value, conventional breeding relies on the transfer and recombination of entire genomes. Desirable genes may therefore be linked, and thus co-inherited, with undesirable genes. Secondly, the sorting and selection of genetically stable new varieties is exceedingly slow. Thirdly, mutations leading to crop improvement occur at very low frequencies, even when artificially induced. Genetic modification offers the opportunity of escaping from each of these limitations.

Putting new genes into plants

Initially, plants proved to be much less amenable than microbes to genetic alteration. Several methods are now available, however, the most widely used being based upon the bacterium *Agrobacterium tumefaciens*, which causes tumours known as crown galls on many flowering plants. This organism contains a tumour-inducing (Ti) plasmid, so-called because galls form when it is transferred to the chromosomes of an infected plant, triggering disorderly growth. Geneticists have now learned to alter the Ti plasmid for their own purposes. By removing its tumour-inducing genes and inserting instead desirable genes taken from bacteria, they have used the plasmid as a vector with which to insert several new genes into plants.

An essential feature of plant genetic modification is the growth of entire plants from single cells. Whereas animal genes not required in a particular tissue are switched off during the course of development, an individual cell from the stem of tobacco, for example, can be cultured to regenerate the entire plant. This process of vegetative propagation is comparable with a gardener taking a cutting from a desirable variety. But the genetic scientist can introduce new genes, allow the cells to proliferate, and then produce thousands of genetically modified plants.

One limitation to Ti plasmid work has been that while *Agrobacterium* infects potatoes, tomatoes, many forest trees, and other dicotyledons, it does not normally attack monocotyledons such as cereals, which are prime targets for genetic improvement. In very recent times, however, this barrier has been circumvented. In addition, alternative methods of gene transfer have emerged. These include the direct introduction of DNA into naked protoplasts—plant cells lacking their tough outer wall, which can be digested away using enzymes. In electroporation, a pulsating electric current is passed through a mixture of protoplasts and DNA. The electrical field opens up tiny pores in the cells, allowing entry of the DNA, which can then be incorporated into the nucleus. Although protoplasts are fragile, the cell wall may grow again within a day or so and the transformed cells can then be cultured to produce whole plants carrying the transferred genes. Sometimes only one in 100,000 protoplasts subsequently divide, however, and not all of these will have taken up and integrated the DNA.

Towards the end of the 1980s, many different research groups were involved in the struggle to bring together in agriculturally important monocotyledons the twin techniques of genetic modification and plant regeneration. There were breakthroughs in using *Agrobacterium* to alter maize and yams genetically, in regenerating rice plants from rice protoplast cultures, and in transforming maize by electroporation (although the resulting plants were infertile). In 1989 maize plants were regenerated from protoplasts (although the technique did not work initially with genetically transformed maize). And in 1990 there was an announcement of fertile maize transformed with a foreign gene that makes the plants resistant to the herbicide Biaphos. In this case the researchers used a 'gene gun' to propel tiny metallic projectiles coated with the relevant genes directly into the cell. They adopted this approach because it allows DNA to be blasted into whole cells—which, unlike protoplasts, have a high likelihood of developing into mature plants. In 1990 too, *Agrobacterium* was used to transform the grapevine genetically for the first time.

Other avenues of plant genetic modification that are now being explored include gene transfer into pollen, and direct injection into reproductive organs. A third emerging possibility is that the jumping genes (transposons) originally discovered by Barbara McClintock may be exploited as tools for genetic modification. As they occur in economically important plants such as maize, it is conceivable that these could be used to ferry into these crops genes for desirable traits such as pest resistance and the capacity to withstand drought.

One experiment designed to assess the behaviour of transposons has acquired historic significance because it was approved in (previously West) Germany in 1989 only after frenetic activity by opponents of genetic modification to prevent 40,000 petunias from being planted out. Researchers at the Max Planck Institute in Cologne had introduced into the petunias a maize gene that turned them an unnatural pink colour. If a transposon were to jump into the middle of this coloration gene, it was likely to leave parts of the flower white. The results should indicate the degree to which transposons move predictably to certain sites or jump more randomly. The study had to take place in the open air because gene jumping was expected to occur in only one out of every 5,000–10,000 petunias, thus necessitating the use of very large numbers of plants. As permission was granted too late for the 1989 growing season, planting took place in 1990.

Somaclonal variation

Plants regenerated from individual cells are not, as was once thought, strictly identical. Because of either subtle differences between the cells of the parent plant, or changes during the culture process, plants produced in this way show considerable differences. This somaclonal variation, although not a form of genetic modification, may provide material from which high-yielding and otherwise desirable varieties can be selected much more quickly than they could be produced by conventional plant breeding—or indeed by recombinant DNA techniques. Unilever scientists have adopted this approach to develop superior oil palms, which contain more oil and a more favourable blend of types of oil. Somaclonal variation has also been used to develop a tomato with an increased content of solids, which is now being used in soups and tomato ketchup. The cells of any one such selected plant *are* identical, so that clones of the chosen type may be cultivated.

Plants with built-in insecticide

As an alternative to using bacteria or viruses as biological insecticides, another option is to incorporate protective genes into plants themselves. Thus researchers at both Monsanto in the USA and Plant Genetic Systems in Belgium have added the toxin gene from *B. thuringiensis* to tobacco, tomato, and other plants and demonstrated that this protects them from destruction by predators. Such **transgenic** plants have enhanced resistance to pests such as butterflies and moths. Tomatoes, for example, can be made resistant to the tobacco hornworm, and to a lesser extent to the tomato fruitworm and the tomato pinworm.

These developments highlight the rival merits of highly specific, as against broad-spectrum, protection. A high degree of specificity between toxin and insect can be seen as a way of fashioning pest resistance which, unlike agrochemical warfare, is capable of being targeted with great accuracy. In other words, it can be seen as much safer simply because it affects only one species, or a very small number of species.

Another approach is to make plants resistant to a wide variety of would-be attackers. One such project began when researchers at the University of Durham were asked to study the heightened tolerance to the bruchid beetle of a particular line of cowpea, Vigna unguiculata, identified at the International Institute for Tropical Agriculture in Nigeria. The biochemical basis of this resistance proved to be elevated levels of an inhibitor of the digestive enzyme trypsin. Several such inhibitors have since been discovered, and are thought to work by interfering with the insect's ability to digest protein.

In association with the Cambridge-based Agricultural Genetics Company, the Durham researchers determined the DNA sequences of a family of four such inhibitors. They then selected a trypsin inhibitor cDNA clone from a cowpea cDNA library, placed it under the control of a gene promoter and transferred it into tobacco cells by using Agrobacterium. Exposed to tobacco budworm, some 20 per cent of the transformed plants showed enhanced resistance. The inserted gene was clearly working well in these plants—the inhibitor amounting to at least 0.5 per cent of the total soluble protein produced in young leaves. The resistance was inherited in a simple Mendelian fashion, and the plants proved resistant to an impressive range of insect pests.

Stealing a virus's clothes

Virus resistance is a key target for plant genetic modification, in view of the enormous economic costs of virus infection. Annual losses in Britain due to viruses attacking potatoes and sugar beet have been estimated at £50m for each crop. In South-East Asia, tungro disease of rice causes losses of some $1,500m per annum, while in Ghana over 190m cocoa trees have been removed since 1946 in efforts to combat cocoa swollen shoot. One approach to the problem is to insert into plant cells the gene coding for the protein that coats a virus particle. Applied to tobacco and the tobacco mosaic virus (TMV), this results in plants that are immune to infection with the virus. When inoculated with TMV, they show no loss of yield, whereas the yields of unmodified plants are reduced by 23–69 per cent.

Similar successes have been reported in making tomato and potato plants resistant to a wide spectrum of viruses, including potato X virus, potato Y virus, alfalfa mosaic virus, and cucumber mosaic virus. The cross-protection is thought to result from interference with the uncoating of virus particles inside the cell before replication.

Herbicide-resistant plants

Another purpose of genetic modification is to develop crops with heightened tolerance to herbicides, such as the selective weed-killers used to prevent broad-leaved plants from growing on lawns. Herbicides are extremely important in agriculture, because they reduce the frequency and thus the cost of tillage to eradicate weeds, boost crop production by reducing competition, and help growers to prevent delays in planting. Crops must, of course, be resistant to the herbicides that are used to protect them, and such tolerance has been a major goal of traditional plant breeding. But there are snags. Several herbicides sprayed on maize in the USA, for example, persist sufficiently to affect soybeans sown the following year. Conventional methods of breeding soybeans with appropriate resistance are limited.

Recombinant DNA techniques allow herbicide-tolerant plants to be created much more quickly and with greater precision. Glyphosate is one commonly used herbicide, which works by blocking an enzyme that is essential for plants to grow. Genes responsible for glyphosate resistance in *E. coli* have been transferred, using *Agrobacterium*, into several plants, including tobacco, rape, and petunia. The plants are able to grow normally even when they are sprayed with the herbicide.

Critics who oppose the development of herbicide-resistant plants argue that their widespread cultivation is likely to increase, rather than decrease, the amounts of chemicals used as herbicides. On the other hand, those who favour this line of research believe that herbicide resistant plants will have the positive impact of reducing overall herbicide use through the substitution of more effective and environmentally acceptable products.

A 'gene-wrecked' tomato

Researchers on opposite sides of the Atlantic–Nottingham University and ICI in the UK, and the Campbell Soup Company and Calgene in the USA—have devised a novel method of preventing fruit from becoming mushy and rotten. Their strategy was to impair the production of polygalac-turonase (PG), the enzyme that normally breaks down the pectin in cell walls and thus softens fruit. The tactics were to interfere with the process of gene transcription by inserting into tomato cells an appropriately synthesized 'anti-sense' piece of DNA, one designed to stick to the messenger RNA for PG and thus prevent it from making PG. Although 10 per cent of PG remained active in early experiments, self-pollination between plants with the highest levels of inhibition produced plants with 99 per cent inhibition of PG. The tomatoes handle better than ordinary tomatoes, and they are said to taste better too. Calgene has registered the 'Flavour Saver Gene' as a trademark.

Nitrogen-fixing plants?

One of the most tempting of all goals for plant genetic modification is to give plants the capacity to fix their own nitrogen from the air, rather than relying on symbiotic rhizobia. This will not be easy, in part because rhizobia require over a dozen different 'nif' genes for nitrogen fixation. Another difficulty is that of persuading the cells of a plant (a eukaryote) to switch on genes transferred from a bacterium (a prokaryote). Although comparable manœuvres have been achieved in cases such as human insulin gene expression in *E. coli*, gene expression following this type of transfer is proving difficult to achieve.

Nutritional Improvement

Another motive for introducing new genes into plants is to raise their nutritional quality. The human body can synthesize only half of the twenty amino acids in protein. Because we must acquire the other ten in our food, it is important that our diet includes adequate quantities of the proteins that can provide these essential substances. The risk of this not happening is all the greater in regions of the world where a single crop provides a major part of the staple diet. In parts of Africa and South America, for example, the proteins in many legumes are low in amino acids containing sulphur. Deficiencies of this sort could be made good by splicing into those crops genes taken from plants, such as the Brazil nut, which have substantial amounts of these amino acids. Similar modifications might be used to raise the contents of oils, fats, and other nutrients.

Medicines from plants

In 1989, US researchers reported that they had transformed tobacco leaf cells by using nucleic acid taken from a mouse hybridoma. This gave the tobacco cells the capacity to produce the same antibodies as those made by the hybridoma cells. There have been other developments too, indicating that plants may be modified and cultivated as factories for making proteins of medical value that are normally produced by animals. Potatoes have been modified to produce serum albumin, a human blood protein that is used to counteract shock and to increase blood volume diminished through surgery or burns. And rape plants have been programmed to produce enkephalin, a natural painkiller synthesized in the human brain. While the production of such substances in microbes represents a major advance over their more painstaking (and occasionally hazardous) extraction from animal tissue, some biotechnologists believe that they can be manufactured even more cheaply in plants.

Can genetically modified plants be released without danger?

The same concerns about the safety of genetically altered microbes disseminated in the environment arise in the case of plants. Although plants could be destroyed by fire or other means if confined in a plot or field, they might well have already been disseminated in the form of pollen, seeds, or other tissues far away from the site of the experiment. Again, assessment of possible hazards rests upon both past experience and a priori reasoning about how a particular plant is likely to behave in a particular environment.

Some scientists cite maize as an example of an invaluable, man-made plant which belies the idea, voiced during the early years of the recombinant DNA debate, that artificially contrived organisms would reproduce uncontrollably. Others argue that the structural changes which have made it dependent upon humans are relatively unusual, and that no overall principles should be drawn from this experience. But there is general agreement that centuries of breeding, carried out with gradually increasing understanding, have not yielded plants capable of causing environmental damage. The fact that even today conventional plant breeding entails gene transfers far more indiscriminate and uncertain than the precise splicing now possible through recombinant DNA techniques, does suggest that such modifications are unlikely to throw up unpredictably hazardous products.

There have, of course, been adverse consequences when certain plants have been disseminated in new terrain either accidentally or purposely but without adequate thought. Salt-cedar, for example, has done considerable damage since it invaded the arid south-western United states earlier this century. Salt-cedar is particularly deep rooted and takes in water at a phenomenal rate. Although the plant requires wet areas for germination and early growth, it can maintain itself on water from deep in the soil once established. Salt-cedar also colonizes natural springs and water courses in desert regions. After invading Eagle Borax Spring in Death Valley during the 1930s, it had caused the total disappearance of surface water from what was once a large marsh by the late 1960s. When the trees were removed, the water returned.

Genetic changes in a plant may also cause ecological changes. One example is the *Spartina anglica* species of cord grass, which originated in the Solent, England, about a century ago. Its ability to grow on barren tidal mudflats has made it into a formidable pest, narrowing waterways and blocking harbours. At the same time, these very qualitites have made the plant a treasured ally when planted to reclaim land and prevent erosion.

Could weeds be made by accident?

One particular hypothetical danger of genetic modification is the accidental production of weeds that grow so aggressively that they obliterate cultivated and other desirable species. This is theoretically possible. But weediness in plants is the consequence of several genes working together, and is thus an unlikely unintended consequence of recombinant DNA modification. As in the case of microbes, decades of experience with plants before the advent of modern gene splicing have also provided a large corpus of knowledge upon which to predict how novel combinations of genes are likely to behave, and how a modified plant will compare with its parents.

Although the accidental production of weeds in the laboratory is unlikely, one question now receiving further study is whether genes are likely to be transferred through pollen from modified plants to relatives which are already weeds. Many of the traits being considered for introduction into crops—for example, herbicide resistance, salt tolerance, and nitrogen fixation —would undoubtedly be beneficial to weeds. Moreover, recent research indicates that pollen can travel further and more quickly than was once thought possible. Likely strategies to prevent the transfer of genes to weedy relatives include measures to promote self-fertilization and to decrease the longevity of pollen.

Aborting normal pollen function

In 1990, Belgian and American scientists applied genetic modification to prevent pollen from developing in tobacco and oilseed rape plants. They added to the plants a gene coding for ribonuclease (an enzyme that breaks down RNA). This was expressed within the anther, selectively destroying the cells lining the pollen sac and thus leading to male sterility. Concurrently, an Australian research group described a naturally occurring system that works in much the same way. The technique will probably be used in future to ensure that farmers plant seed obtained by crossing two parent lines of maize, for example, which they are certain will give high-yielding hybrids, rather than seed derived from self-pollination or random pollination. At present, laborious (and expensive) hand emasculation has to be used to produce hybrid seeds of maize, tomato, cabbage, and other crop plants. Similar methods of inducing sterility might also be exploited to ensure that introduced genes are not disseminated through the pollen of genetically modified plants.

Chapter Seven

Genetic Modification and Animals

Animal breeding today

Science has brought three major advances in animal husbandry in recent years, extending, simplifying, and speeding up the breeding of high quality farm animals. First, ordinary commercial females such as cows and ewes can now serve as surrogate mothers for the rearing of embryos from pedigree breeding stock. The initial step in this process is to give hormones to high quality females, inducing multiple ovulation. The ova are fertilized (either in the dam herself or in the test-tube) with sperm from high quality males. The resulting embryos are then transferred into surrogates. Applied to dairy stock, this technique enables a top quality cow to produce as many as 20, rather than an average of 3.5, daughters per lifetime. The same approach is also used to breed special lines of both sheep and cattle for enhanced meat production. Secondly, embryos can be frozen for storage and transportation, making breeding programmes very much more flexible than they were hitherto. In North America alone, over 100,000 cows per year now receive embryos from other cows, and many of these come from frozen embryos. Importation of frozen embryos is also a more economical way of making high quality breeds available to countries that could not otherwise afford them. Thirdly, pedigree livestock can be cloned, giving large numbers of genetically identical animals with superior milk- or meat-producing capabilities. This does not mean the production of copies of a particular adult animal, but the cloning of embryos. One technique is to split an embryo into two parts, which are then implanted and continue to develop as they would have done as a whole. Two or at most four identical calves can be produced in this way.

The alternative technique involves nuclear transfer which resets the clock of development. A technician, using microsurgical equipment, separates an eight- or sixteen-cell embryo into its individual cells and removes their nuclei. Each nucleus is then placed into a single-cell, newly fertilized egg, whose own nucleus has been removed. The cells are then transferred to foster mothers. Although not all may develop to term, several genetically identical calves and sheep can be produced in this way (see Fig. 7.1). The precise quality of such a clone of animals can not, of course, be known in advance. The strategy now emerging, therefore, is to implant one or two of the modified cells into a foster mother and to assess the milk or meat production of the resulting animal when it grows to maturity. The remaining cells, frozen meanwhile, can then be implanted and used for further, limitless rounds of cloning.

In a variant on this second strategy, now under development, the nuclei are taken from the inner mass of **stem cells** in an embryo. Because these cells retain their capacity to divide but do not differentiate, they provide an unlimited source of nuclei for nuclear transfer. For all practical purposes, this could mean virtually no limit on the number of animals that could be cloned from a pedigree animal.

These are dramatic advances. Even more spectacular is the production of chimaeras containing the cells of two distinct animals such as sheep and goats. But all of these developments are based on the modification of cells, not on the transfer of genes. They stem from research centred on the idea of optimizing our use of existing species of animal rather than fabricating novel ones. Now, however, we stand on the threshold of an era in which transgenic animals containing genes from other species could be widely used in agriculture and other fields.

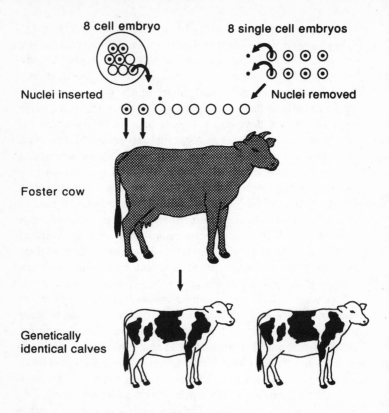

Fig. 7.1 Cloning calves by nuclear transfer

Mixing cells rather than mixing genes

Genetic modification in animals should not be confused with the production of chimaeras. Chimaeras occur naturally in cattle, as a consequence of non-identical twins sharing the same placenta. A few years ago, however, researchers at the then Agricultural Research Council Institute of Animal Physiology in Cambridge set out to produce artificial chimaeras between sheep and goats. Previous work had shown that the transfer of embryos from one to the other induced early pregnancy. But the embryos did not survive for more than a week's gestation, probably as a result of immunological rejection. Could this incompatibility be surmounted by producing embryonic sheep–goat chimaeras and transferring them from one animal to another?

The Cambridge group carried out three different sets of experiments. First they took individual blastomeres (cells produced during cleavage) from four-cell goat embryos. They then combined them with blastomeres from either four- or eight-cell sheep embryos. In each case the mixture was enveloped within a zona pellucida—the normal outer membrane of the egg, evacuated for this purpose. Second, they wrapped blastomeres taken from eight-cell sheep embryos around an eight-cell goat embryo from which they had removed the zona pellucida. They also did the reverse, surrounding a similarly denuded sheep embryo with blastomeres separated from a goat embryo. Composite embryos from the first two types of experiment were embedded in agar and grown for several days inside sheeps' oviducts. The researchers then examined them, and transferred those which had become normal-looking blastocysts into either ewes or goats on the seventh day of the oestrous cycle.

Older materials—the so-called inner cell mass and polar trophectoderm from eight-day-old goat blastocysts—were used for the third group of modifications. The researchers inserted these into sheep blastocysts of the same age, and also carried out the opposite manœuvre, transferring the products into either sheep or goats on the eighth day of their cycle. Judging by the outcome of those pregnancies in all three types of experiment which had a successful culmination, three things became clear. Sheep and goat blastomeres can unite to form viable blastocysts. They contain the cells of both species, and may give rise to animals that are genuine sheep–goat chimaeras. Three of the seven young born as a result of the first experiments—all looking like lambs—had bands of hair, contrasting with densely curled wool in the rest of the fleece. Two had a twin, with ordinary wool, produced from the same two parent embryos. The researchers concluded that the hairy bands were goat tissue and that the creatures were chimaeras. Likewise, one of the young from the second group of experiments resembled an ordinary kid, except that some of its goat hair was replaced by densely curled wool.

Similar chimaeras were produced as a result of the third set of modifications. Six of the nine young looked in every respect like lambs. But of the remaining three, one resembled the chimaeric lambs in the first experiments. Another seemed very much like the chimaeric kid produced in the second series, except that its skin had bands of wool along the back. Other offspring appeared to be quite ordinary kids—though one, born as a twin to one of the kids, looked like a lamb.

The research team concluded that the third series of experiments indicates that in sheep and goats it is possible to neutralize completely incompatibility between the conceptus and the recipient female. This had been achieved by constructing the chimaeric embryo in such a way that the trophectoderm and hence the chorionic epithelium consisted entirely of cells belonging to the same species as the recipient.

The real breakthrough from this work was not chimaera production for its own sake, but knowledge of how to persuade one genus of animal to carry to term a fetus of another genus. Many animals around the world, such as the European Bison, have lost their wildland habitats and are being kept alive solely in zoos. The habitats of many more are now threatened. Removal of natural barriers to reproduction could be a great advantage to conservationists in breeding rare species.

Transgenic animals

Genetic modification in animals has followed its application in microbes and plants. Foreign genes (which must, of course, be accompanied by the appropriate regulatory sequences) can now be introduced into, and be expressed in, animal cells. If a gene is to be present in all of the cells of an animal, including the germ cells, it must be introduced at a very early stage in development. This can be done by giving hormones to encourage a female to superovulate, providing a large supply of eggs. The eggs are then fertilized and each one is immobilized under a microscope and injected with a solution of cloned DNA directly into one of the two pronuclei it contains. Each of these pronuclei (one derived from the egg cell and the other from the fertilizing spermatozoon) contains the haploid number (i.e. one set) of chromosomes. In a proportion of cases, the injected DNA integrates into one or more of the chromosomes, usually as a long head-to-tail array comprising many copies of the DNA fragment. Modified embryos are transferred to a foster mother and the resulting offspring can then be screened for the presence of the foreign gene (see Fig. 7.2).

Although this technique of pronuclear injection remains the most widely used method of genetic modification in animals, two other approaches are finding increasing favour because they can position the new gene more precisely in its new setting. The first technique is to transfer DNA into embryonic stem cells—cell lines which are derived from preimplantation embryos and can be grown indefinitely in the test-tube. Cells that express the introduced DNA (i.e. they produce the relevant protein) can be selected in the test-tube and be injected into the blastocoel cavity of a normal embryo and thence be transferred into a foster mother.

The immediate offspring following this type of modification will be **mosaics**, some of the cells in various organs (including the gonads) being genetically altered cells. However, breeding from this generation leads to segregation of the introduced gene, so that a proportion of the next generation consists of completely transgenic animals. The opportunity to manipulate and select cells in the test-tube means that a gene may, if the sequence is known, be targeted at a specific site in the chromosome.

Another method is to exploit retroviruses as vectors to ferry

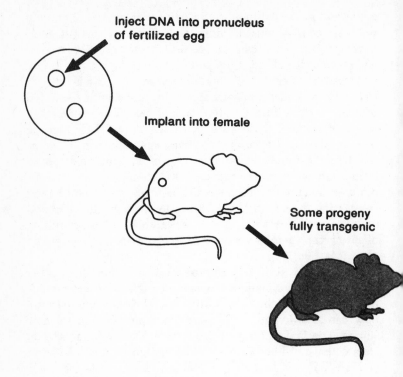

Fig. 7.2 Producing transgenic mice

new genes into animal cells. By replacing a retrovirus's own genes (leaving only the so-called long terminal repeats at each end) with an RNA version of a cloned gene, one can ensure that its DNA copy is integrated into the chromosomes of the animal cell. Normally only a single copy of the gene is integrated into the cell. Moreover, the virus cannot replicate itself because it now lacks the requisite genes. Retrovirus vectors (which can carry only relatively short sequences) may be introduced into preimplantation embryos in a variety of different ways. Again, the offspring will consist of a mosaic of normal and transgenic cells.

Pharmaceutical farming

One of the applications of transgenic livestock could be to produce rare and expensive proteins for use in human medicine. This can be achieved, for example, by linking the gene coding for a particular protein to a promoter which ensures that the gene is expressed only in the sheep mammary gland. The protein can then be recovered from the animal's milk. Researchers in Edinburgh have already used this approach to arrange for the sheep to secrete in their milk the blood clotting protein known as factor IX (lack of which causes one type of haemophilia). They inserted the new gene alongside the regulatory region of the lactoglobulin gene, which encodes one of the proteins in sheep's milk, by injection into fertilized eggs.

The same strategy has been adopted to produce alpha-1-antitrypsin, deficiency of which results in emphysema. Other pharmaceuticals that have already been made in animals in small-scale experiments include tissue plasminogen activator in goats, interleukin-2 in rabbits, and human growth hormone in mice.

Although the yields of proteins produced in these experiments were at first lower than anticipated, these have now been improved and some research workers believe that many different pharmaceuticals can be made more cheaply in transgenic animals than by other methods. Proteins obtained in this way are purified by spinning out the milk fat in a centrifuge, precipitating the proteins, and subjecting them to chromatography. This gives products as pure as those made by culturing microbial cells and purer than when factor IX, for example, is obtained by extracting it from blood. The proponents of this method of manufacture argue that the cost of a flock of, say, 2,000 transgenic milking sheep would be modest as compared with that of fermentation equipment with the same output of a particular protein. They also point to the greater evolutionary affinity between humans and these mammalian producers, as compared with cultures of bacteria.

Many human proteins are glycosylated—they have sugar molecules attached to them. Proteins made in bacteria lack these sugars, which can mean that they are more rapidly eliminated from the body after injection.

Transgenic animals as models of disease

Another protein that has been produced in transgenic animals (in mice) is human haemoglobin. In this case, the aim was not to make haemoglobin for therapeutic use. It was to develop an animal model that can be used to study diseases such as sickle cell anaemia which are characterized by the formation of abnormal types of haemoglobin. Similarly, research into cancer is benefiting from the development of oncomice whose hereditary material includes genes predisposing them to develop cancer. The first of these to be introduced—and the first genetically altered animal to be patented—was a mouse carrying the 'ras' oncogene that is common in a variety of human cancers. It also carries a mouse mammary tumour virus promoter, which ensures that the oncogene is activated in breast tissue. As a result, the mice develop a human breast cancer within a few months of birth. Produced by Harvard University in collaboration with the chemical company, the Du Pont Corporation, and patented in the USA in 1988, this and other oncomice are used to test drugs against human cancers. They are also valuable for research into the molecular biology of cancer.

Boosting agricultural productivity

Two different approaches have been developed to enhance the productivity of livestock. One approach makes use of bacteria to clone the gene for the growth hormone—bovine somatotropin (BST). The hormone is then injected into dairy cows to increase their milk yield. BST injections can also be given to reduce the amount of fat in pigs and other meat animals. The second approach is to produce transgenic livestock carrying the bovine or human growth hormone gene. Experiments of this sort have shown reduced fat deposits and increased wool growth. But they have also led to severe side-effects such as arthritis, gastric ulcers, and infertility in pigs carrying the bovine growth hormone gene.

Promoting disease resistance

The arrival of transgenic technology has stimulated renewed interest in the genes responsible for resistance against particular disease. Such genes might be cloned and introduced into otherwise vulnerable breeds of animal, to protect them against those conditions. One example is the genes that control the incubation period of scrapie, thereby making some breeds of sheep far less susceptible to this wasting disease, which is caused by a prion. Another example is the genes conferring the natural resistance to trypanosomiasis that is found in certain breeds of cattle. Introducing genes of this type into breeds that are already desirable in other ways could have important consequences for animal husbandry.

Correcting genetic disorders

Recent research with transgenic animals has pointed the way towards the correction of one particular genetic defect. Working with mouse stem cells, scientists in Edinburgh selected cells with a mutation in the gene for the production of an enzyme called hypoxanthine phosphoribosyltransferase (HPRT). When these cells were introduced into mouse embryos and transferred to foster mothers, some of the offspring were totally deficient in HPRT. But the deficiency could be corrected by inserting an HPRT gene into the stem cells. This was the first ever demonstration that a precise genetic alteration could be introduced into a mammal's germ line. In humans, absence of HPRT results in the severe and usually fatal Lesch-Nyhan syndrome. Although this work is of relevance to the human syndrome, any hopes of treatment for the condition are still many years away. It would not be possible to treat patients by somatic cell gene therapy, and genetic intervention in human germ cells is not currently on the agenda for both practical and ethical reasons.

From fish to mosquitoes

Two final examples illustrate the potential range and diversity of animal genetic modification. One, the genetic modification of fish, is now becoming established commercially. The other, the production of transgenic mosquitoes, remains a promising avenue of research.

In one sense, fish eggs are easier to manipulate than their mammalian counterparts, because they are large, plentiful, and do not have to be transferred back into the mother after fertilization. But the eggs of some species of fish are surrounded by very tough outer membranes. Chemical and other techniques have had to be developed to disrupt this barrier and allow foreign DNA inside. Fish too have a growth hormone, production of which could in principle be harnessed to improve growth rate and productivity. Yearling rainbow trout have been found to grow twice as quickly when injected with the hormone. The hormone was made by taking growth hormone messenger RNA from trout pituitary glands, making the corresponding DNA sequence and inserting it into bacteria. More recently, the gene coding for the hormone has been a major target for genetic modification. When the gene for either fish growth hormone or bovine growth hormone is incorporated into loach or goldfish, they grow up to four times faster than normal.

Mosquitoes are targets for genetic modification because of possible benefits in the world-wide battle against insect-borne disease. One technique used with limited success to attack mosquito populations in the past was to release massive numbers of sterile males. These would compete with natural fertile males for female partners and thus reduce the numbers of offspring. But the relatively crude chemical and other methods which were then used to induce sterility also seemed to impair the mosquitoes' reproductive competitiveness. There are now hopes that much more subtle genetic changes can be made, resulting in males that are sterile but vigorous in their sexual advances!

Genes into muscle and other cells

In the next chapter we shall be considering progress towards gene therapy in human patients—the alteration of human genes to ameliorate disease. The most likely early steps in this direction will probably involve making genetic changes to abnormal cells in particular tissues. In 1990, US scientists reported studies in mice that indicate one possible approach. They injected DNA coding for three different enzymes into the muscles of live mice, and found that the genes were expressed just as effectively as when the DNA was added to cells in a test tube. Around the same time, the team at Duke University in North Carolina which developed the 'gene gun' for propelling DNA directly into plant cells announced that it had modified the technique to insert genes into a wide variety of organs in living mice. Genes spliced into plasmids and then blasted into muscle, liver, spleen, and intestinal cells were expressed in those tissues. Although the plasmids were designed not to replicate themselves in their new setting, the genes worked for up to three weeks in the liver cells. The genes inserted in this way were those coding for human growth hormone and luciferase, the enzyme that is responsible for luminescence in fireflies. The researchers reported that the animals suffered no trauma or irritation to the skin as a result of the procedure.

Making proteins to order—monoclonal antibodies

As we saw earlier, genetic modification has been used to alter the structure of proteins—to make enzymes more resistant to heat, for example. Paralleling that sort of application has been an innovation in the production of another type of protein—

extremely pure monoclonal antibodies, which have brought dramatic changes in biological research and medical diagnosis. In this case, the process begins not with recombinant DNA research but with the immunization of animals. However, research is now moving towards the possibility that such antibodies can be made to order without using animals at all.

An antibody is a Y-shaped molecule consisting of two heavy and two light chains of amino acids. At the tips of the arms are the so-called variable domains, whose amino acid sequences recognize and match particular antigens. The sequences in the remainder of the antibody—the trunk—are relatively constant and common to all antibodies produced by a particular animal. Their task is to engage defensive mechanisms such as the gobbling up by phagocytes of invading organisms whose antigens betray their foreignness (see Fig. 7.3).

Monoclonal antibodies are produced by hybridomas, which were developed by the Argentinian-British molecular biologist,

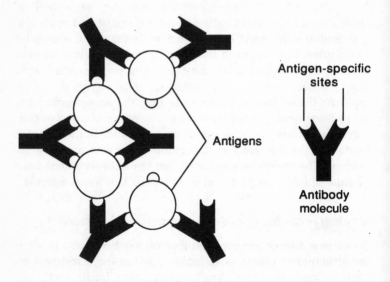

Fig. 7.3 Antibodies and antigens

Milstein, and the West German molecular biologist, Kohler, when they were working together at the Medical Research Council Laboratories in Cambridge. They injected mice with an antigen, inducing certain white blood cells to generate the corresponding antibody. They then took some of these cells and fused them in laboratory glassware with malignant cells. The resulting hybridomas combined the antibody-making capacity of white cells with the immortality of malignant cells (which, unlike normal cells, grow indefinitely when cultured in the laboratory). Individual hybridoma cells could then be cultured to yield clones of identical cells. Grown in massive quantities, these could provide limitless amounts of specific antibodies.

Applications of monoclonal antibodies hinge upon their propensity to recognize and latch on to corresponding antigens—usually proteins on the surface of cells. They range from blood typing and the identification of infectious agents (especially when present in tiny quantities) to the purification of products such as interferon after they have been made by genetically modified microbes. Their capacity to home in on specific antigens, including those that characterize certain cancer cells, suggests that monoclonal antibodies might also be exploited to direct toxic drugs onto particular targets in malignant tissue.

The possibility of supplanting animals altogether in the production of antibodies arises from further recent research by Greg Winter and his collaborators in Cambridge. This indicates that effective antibodies can be made in bacteria programmed with the appropriate gene. The Cambridge researchers have already inserted into a bacteriophage a gene specifying an antibody that recognizes a protein called lysozyme, and demonstrated that when bacteria are infected with the phage they begin to produce that antibody. Large libraries of antibody genes might be created in this way, allowing antibodies to be made to order in bacteria. Although such genes would have to be obtained originally from animal cells, they could be modified and exploited thereafter in bacteria.

Because the genes coding for the different domains of an antibody can be cut and spliced together, chimaeric antibodies may be produced. For example, the variable domains of a mouse antibody directed against a particular microbe can be attached to the constant domains of human antibody. Given to a human patient to combat an infection with that organism, such an antibody would be less likely to provoke immune rejection by the human body than a wholly mouse antibody.

Greg Winter and his colleagues have taken this principle further. They have linked the discrete binding site only (rather than the entire variable domain) from an antibody produced in one species to the constant domains of antibody from another species. One application was to reshape an antibody made by immunizing rats with a particular type of human white blood cells, which is used to treat certain forms of cancer. When the Cambridge researchers 'humanized' the rat antibodies by hooking up their binding sites to constant domains of human antibodies, the resulting antibodies were more effective than the complete rat antibody when used to treat a human lymphoma. Antibodies of this sort are even less likely than chimaeric antibodies to be rejected by immune defence mechanisms.

Single domain antibodies

Another recent development in Winter's laboratory is the surprising discovery that many isolated variable regions of the heavy chain can bind antigens in the absence of their light chain partners. These mini-antibodies, which have been called single domain antibodies, can be produced in the bacterium *E. coli*. A mouse is immunized against a particular antigen, and DNA is extracted from antibody-producing cells in the animal's spleen. The polymerase chain reaction is then used to amplify DNA fragments which are transferred into and expressed in *E. coli*. Colonies of the bacterium are screened to find those producing single domain antibodies. The whole process is remarkably quick. Single domain antibodies can be generated within days, as compared with a month or so when hybridomas are used to make monoclonal antibodies. Another advantage is a considerable reduction in the number of animals required.

Single domain antibodies are expected to rival monoclonals in applications such as diagnosis, the purification of proteins, the ridding of toxins from the body, and the tissue targeting of toxins as magic bullets. Because they are composed of much smaller molecules, they should also be able to penetrate infected and malignant tissues more readily, and reach 'deep canyon sites' on viruses.

There are strong parallels between the binding of a particular antibody to its corresponding antigen and the binding of an enzyme to the substrate(s) it is about to transform. Recognition of this similarity has led to the production of monoclonal antibodies that resemble enzymes in catalysing chemical changes. These abzymes have been shown to be capable of actions such as cutting through the protein coat of viruses and detoxifying poisonous chemicals.

Chapter Eight

Genetic Screening and Gene Therapy in People

Preventing human genetic disorders

Thousands of human illnesses have been traced to defective genes. Many of them are serious and distressing conditions. Many cannot be cured or even treated directly—as a bacterial infection can be attacked by an antibiotic. At most, some of the symptoms can be relieved. For example, the build-up of mucus that is associated with cystic fibrosis can be ameliorated—but only by frequent and painful physiotherapy. A major goal of current research is that such conditions may be dealt with by **gene therapy**—by replacing or repairing the malfunctioning gene. This could be achieved, not by interfering with DNA in egg cells or spermatozoa (germ-line gene therapy), as in the production of transgenic animals, but by altering genes in particular tissues of the body (somatic cell gene therapy).

Germ-line gene therapy is not considered a legitimate target for human medicine, at least in the foreseeable future. While it could offer the prospect of removing a serious inherited disease from a family, therapy of this sort raises serious ethical issues. Moreover, it is unnecessary as preimplantation diagnosis and embryo selection achieves the same end, more simply and safely. In principle, the goal of somatic cell gene therapy is to overcome congenital disease caused by defects in genes whose normal functions are to produce particular enzymes or other proteins. One example is thalassaemia, which occurs when bone marrow cells destined to become red blood cells fail to produce sufficient quantities of haemoglobin. This happens because of a defect in one of the major globin genes. Here and in the case of genetic defects in other tissues, the objective would be to reinstate the capacity to produce the missing protein by correcting or compensating for the underlying genetic defect.

Somatic cell gene therapy would help only the individual being treated. Germ-line gene therapy, on the other hand, would correct the genetic defect in the germ cells, thereby preventing the disease in future generations. A fully functional gene would be introduced into the fertilized egg cell or very early embryo ensuring that it was replicated as cells divided and thus present in virtually all of the cells of the fully grown individual. Any mistake in germ-line gene therapy might lead to the corresponding aberration appearing in every cell of the adult in due course.

The year 1990 saw the announcement of the first concrete steps in human somatic cell gene therapy. These advances have emerged from a wider programme of research on the mapping and screening of genetic defects. Therefore, before discussing gene therapy, which has generated so much attention, it is appropriate to consider an approach which is already reducing the burden of suffering caused by cystic fibrosis, the thalassaemias, Duchenne muscular dystrophy, and other genetic disorders.

The first part of this two-part approach is to locate the genes responsible for such conditions, or at least marker genes closely linked to the gene concerned. The second is to screen fetal cells early in pregnancy for those labels (pre-natal screening). Combined together, these techniques make it possible to identify affected embryos, and thus to prevent disease by terminating the pregnancy if the couple concerned chooses. We shall begin with pre-natal screening because these methods are more fully developed than the ability to locate disease-causing genes and because they provide useful information even before the specific DNA sequences responsible for particular diseases have been pinpointed.

Pre-natal screening

In situations in which there is a family history of a Mendelian disorder or inherited chromosomal abnormality, when a couple already have a defective child, or when the mother is over 35 (and therefore more likely to give birth to a child with Down's syndrome), pre-natal diagnosis is usually offered. It can provide results that either reassure the parents or give them information on which they can make a decision on whether or not to terminate the pregnancy.

Amniocentesis is a well-established method of pre-natal diagnosis, which is carried out at 15–16 weeks gestation. Ultrasound scanning is used to locate the placenta, and a small quantity of amniotic fluid is withdrawn through a needle from the amniotic cavity. In addition to chemical analysis of the fluid for substances indicative of conditions such as spina bifida, amniotic cells (which have been shed from the skin of the fetus) can be cultured and their chromosomes examined to confirm or exclude Down's syndrome. The amniotic fluid also provides DNA which can be studied to reveal the increasing number of recognized inborn errors of metabolism and other genetically based conditions.

Chorionic villus sampling (CVS), introduced more recently, performs the same function as amniocentesis. However, it has a significant advantage over amniocentesis in that the procedure can be carried out appreciably earlier, in the first trimester of pregnancy, with both clinical and psychological benefits if a termination should be decided upon. Chorionic villi are part of the developing placenta, and can be removed using an aspiration needle, either through the vagina or through the abdomen, as early as 8 weeks and up to 11 or 12 weeks. Because the cells of the chorionic villus are derived from the fertilized egg, they are able to provide a reliable guide to the genetic constitution of the fetus. One disadvantage of CVS, however, is that it is associated with a higher spontaneous abortion rate than that associated with amniocentesis. Amniocentesis increases the risk of miscarriage by about 1 per cent whereas CVS increases it by about 4 per cent.

The sex of a fetus can also be determined by analysing cells obtained using either of these techniques. Although parents could exploit the results to choose the sex of their offspring for non-medical reasons, the principal purpose is to help them decide on termination if the mother is likely to give birth to a child affected by a condition determined by one of the sex chromosomes. In certain disorders associated with an abnormal gene carried on the X chromosome, for example, knowledge of the sex of a fetus may be useful when a more specific test (of the sort outlined in the next section) is not available.

Probes, markers, and other revealing methods

Linkage analysis, based on the extent to which particular genes are inherited together, allows the positions of mutant genes responsible for certain inherited conditions to be located on the human chromosomes. The technique requires several generations and large numbers of individuals, and is thus much more difficult when applied to humans rather than to *Drosophila* or pea plants. Nevertheless, many genes have been located in this way and then cloned and their DNA sequences determined. This makes it possible to produce corresponding DNA probes, which facilitate conclusive identification.

Many other disorders, whose genes have not yet been isolated, have been mapped to their approximate chromosomal locations. These genes too can be identified by using linked DNA markers, although with less certainty. By the end of the century, it is intended that the positions of all human genes will be known, and all clinically important genes will have been sequenced, through the Human Genome Project.

Screening for haemoglobin disorders

The World Health Organization forecasts that by the year 2000 approximately 7 per cent of the world's population will be carriers of the most important haemoglobinopathies. These are serious conditions, caused by a failure of haemoglobin, found in red blood cells, to carry oxygen to the tissues in the normal way. They are the commonest of all genetic disorders in people. Because methods of treatment are far from satisfactory, the current approach is to try to avoid the birth of affected children. Pre-natal diagnosis followed by termination of pregnancy and the detection of carriers will therefore remain the principal means of combating these disorders in the foreseeable future.

In some disorders, such as sickle cell anaemia, an abnormality in the structure of the haemoglobin molecule is to blame. Thalassaemias, on the other hand, occur when one or more of the four globin chains (two alpha, two beta) comprising the molecule are produced at a diminished rate, leading to an imbalance in their proportions. In alpha thalassaemia, production of alpha globin chains is either absent (alpha^0) or reduced (alpha$^+$). Both alpha globin genes are deleted from one chromosome in individuals with the alpha^0 thalassaemia trait (all four being deleted in the homozygous state). Only one alpha globin gene is inactivated (by deletion or mutation) in the alpha$^+$ thalassaemia trait, the other remaining intact. Over 90 different mutations have been found to cause beta thalassaemia. They either prevent (beta^0) or diminish (beta$^+$) the formation of beta globin chains. Note that while such mutations differ one from another (producing different genotypes) the end-result (the phenotype) can be exactly the same.

Considerable advances have been made in recent years in the pre-natal diagnosis of haemoglobinopathies, much of the work being pioneered by Sir David Weatherall and his colleagues at the John Radcliffe Hospital, Oxford. These advances in genetic diagnosis have built upon earlier techniques that identified abnormal forms of the haemoglobin in red blood cells, obtained by passing a needle into the placenta or umbilical cord and withdrawing blood. Although these methods were effective (resulting in, for example, a marked fall in the birth rate of beta thalassaemia homozygotes in Cyprus), they had the great disadvantage that they could not be used until late in the second trimester of pregnancy. Focusing on genes, rather than on the haemoglobins they produce, the newer approaches can be adopted before blood cells are available for sampling. The first such advances, in the late 1970s, were made using amniotic fluid cells obtained early in the second trimester. The first successful diagnoses on DNA in chorionic villi, sampled late in the first trimester, occurred during the early 1980s.

When a specific gene probe is available, pre-natal diagnosis is relatively simple. Sickle cell anaemia, which is caused by the substitution of one amino acid, glutamic acid, by valine at a particular position in the beta globin chain, illustrates the principle. This disorder can be diagnosed by detecting the mutation concerned in chorionic villus cells. A technician extracts DNA from the cells and then adds a restriction endonuclease that cuts the gene at the codon for glutamic acid. The DNA 'digest' is then placed on a gel to separate different sized fragments and is treated with a labelled probe for the globin gene. A film then reveals the result. If the haemoglobin is normal, the endonuclease will have split it into two pieces, each of which hybridizes with the probe. This produces two dark bands. If the haemoglobin is of the sickle cell variety, it will not have been split and there will thus be only one dark band (see Fig. 8.1).

In the case of alpha thalassaemia, failure of hybridization with alpha globin gene probes can also be used to demonstrate gene deletion in the homozygous state. But in most of the haemoglobinopathies, diagnosis rests upon the identification of **restriction fragment length polymorphisms (RFLP)**. Because of the number of mutations involved, beta thalassaemia is a more difficult proposition. If DNA analysis is to be used for pre-natal diagnosis, each individual family has to be studied to determine the nature of the mutation—although certain specific probes are useful in populations where particular mutations are common.

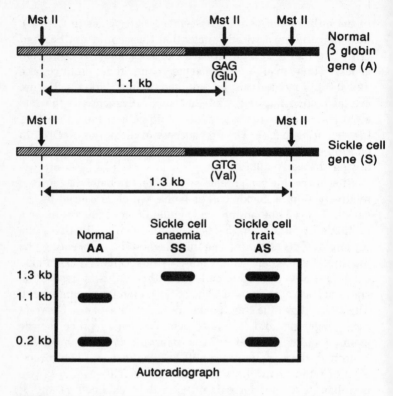

Fig. 8.1 Pre-natal diagnosis of sickle cell anaemia using the restriction enzyme Mst II

In Sardinia, for example, where the majority of cases of beta thalassaemia result from a nonsense mutation at a specific position on the beta chain gene, one research group has reported using a particular gene probe to identify 94 couples out of 193 pregnancies at risk for carrying a fetus homozygous for beta⁰ thalassaemia who had this mutation. In a country such as the UK, where the immigrant population at risk of haemoglobin disorders is drawn from the Mediterranean region, the Indian subcontinent, the Middle East, and elsewhere, and contains individuals with a wide range of different thalassaemia mutations, the task of pre-natal diagnosis and screening is much more challenging.

Pre-natal diagnosis using restriction fragment length polymorphisms (RFLPs)

When a specific gene probe is available, as for sickle cell disease, pre-natal diagnosis is relatively straightforward. However, a quite different screening tactic is necessary in the case of Huntington's disease. This is a progressive affliction of the central nervous system, characterized by involuntary movements, loss of motor control, and dementia. The symptoms usually appear in the fourth or fifth decade of life. There is no cure. Nothing other than symptomatic treatment is possible, and the symptoms progress until the patient dies 15–17 years later. Huntington's disease is inherited as a dominant trait which means that every son and daughter of an affected person has a 50 per cent chance of developing the condition.

Pre-natal diagnosis of Huntington's disease rests upon a technique, devised in the late 1970s, which greatly accelerated the speed at which human genes could be mapped. This technique makes ingenious use of differences (polymorphisms) in non-coding DNA sequences that can be found littered throughout the human chromosomes. Some of these differences, which are known as restriction fragment length polymorphisms, occur at the sites that are cut by restriction enzymes.

A given piece of DNA, broken up by enzymes, produces a distinctive set of fragments. These can be separated (by electrophoresis) to produce a pattern similar to that of a bar code. DNA from an early embryo or a child or adult can therefore be compared with DNA from normal and affected members of a family to determine which cutting sites are associated with mutant genes and which with normal genes. If the DNA in question produces the same pattern as that of affected family members, then the chances are high that the aberrant gene occurs in the cells from which it came (see Fig. 8.2). (The RFLP bar codes cannot be generalized as the basis for a universal test because although the cutting sites are the same within a family, they differ from one family to another.)

Some years ago, researchers found an RFLP on chromosome number 4 that was linked to the Huntington's disease locus. Investigators can, therefore, determine which RFLP pattern segregates with the disease by analysing DNA samples from both affected and elderly unaffected individuals in a family. At risk persons can then be tested to determine whether they have that RFLP. Because the marker is some distance from the gene, the test is only about 95 per cent accurate, although the reliability of more recently discovered markers is up to 99 per cent. The test is usually offered to couples prior to pregnancy in order to provide family members with the information they need to help make decisions for the future and reproductive choices.

The cystic fibrosis gene—a screening dilemma

In 1989, researchers at the Hospital for Sick Children, Toronto, and the universities of Toronto and Michigan announced that they had located the mutant gene responsible for cystic fibrosis (CF). This was a triumph for Lap-Chee Tsui and Francis Collins and their co-workers in their use of the elegant but nevertheless laborious techniques of reverse genetics. First, they studied members of families with the disease, and used linkage analysis to locate the gene on chromosome 7. Then they sought further genetic markers, one on either side of the target gene, which were inherited along with the CF gene in affected families. After locating two that were still a considerable distance apart, they examined another 250 such markers and found two which they thought were inside the earlier pair and thus closer to the CF gene.

At this point, the Toronto researchers adopted a technique known as chromosome walking—cloning all of the sequences

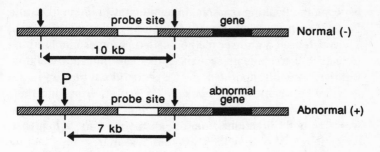

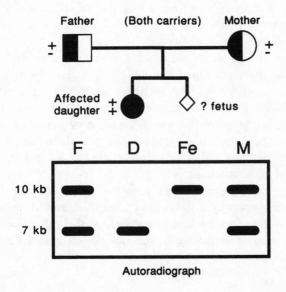

Fig. 8.2 Pre-natal diagnosis of a recessive disorder using restriction fragment length polymorphism (RFLP) linkage analysis

Note: P indicates a polymorphic restriction enzyme site. The autoradiograph shows that the fetus is normal

between the flanking markers, in an attempt to home in on the target. This process must result in cloning of the required gene. They also used a quicker method called chromosome jumping to leap over unclonable sequences that can interrupt walking. But they were disappointed: the CF gene did not turn up in the territory between the two markers. So Tsui, Collins, and their co-workers began walking and jumping again, moving outwards in both directions from one of the markers. When they encountered a gene which another research group, led by Robert Williamson at St Mary's Hospital, London, had already found to be closely linked with the CF gene, they knew they were progressing in the right direction. Final success came when they found a gene with a sequence that matched the sequence of DNA copied from a fragment of messenger RNA isolated from sweat gland cells—one of the types of cell in which the CF gene is expressed.

The Toronto discovery led quickly to the development of a DNA probe specific for the CF mutation. As well as being used in affected families, this seemed likely to be taken up quickly as the basis for major screening programmes in whole populations. These hopes were dimmed, however, when the newly identified mutant gene was found in only about 75 per cent of CF patients. Other mutations (possibly a considerable number of different ones) seemed to be responsible for the remaining cases. Since 1989 some of these further CF-predisposing mutations have been identified and it is now possible to detect 84 per cent of carriers. At this rate of carrier detection general screening of the population may be more feasible.

Neurofibromatosis—another cloning triumph

Mapping and cloning techniques, similar to those deployed against the cystic fibrosis gene, provided another breakthrough in 1990 when US scientists announced the discovery of the gene that causes neurofibromatosis. Characterized by numerous benign tumours, learning disabilities, and other neurological symptoms, this is the disorder popularly though erroneously associated with the name of Joseph Merrick, the 'Elephant Man'. The gene proved to be huge, anywhere from half a million to two million bases long. It also has at least three other genes buried within it—only the second 'megagene' ever to have been found with other gene sequences nested within it. In this case, identification of the gene seems unlikely to lead to a screening test that can be widely applied, because researchers have found a different mutation in almost every affected family where the genetic defect itself, rather than a linked genetic marker, has been identified. Moreover, half of the cases of neurofibromatosis arise not from an inherited mutant gene but from a new, spontaneous mutation that has occurred for the first time in the affected individual.

Screening IVF embryos

In 1989, there was a major development in screening for genetic defects in cells derived from preimplantation embryos produced by *in vitro* fertilization (that is, by adding spermatozoa to egg cells growing in laboratory glassware). This technique is aimed at couples at high risk of producing a baby suffering from a severe genetic disease and would allow unaffected embryos to be selected and implanted in the woman, who would then be assured that her pregnancy would be free of any risk from that particular inherited disorder.

Robert Winston and colleagues in London reported that they had been able to remove single cells from very early (6–10 cell) human embryos and then to sex them by using the polymerase chain reaction (PCR) to amplify a repeated sequence specific to the Y chromosome. Removal of a single cell from an embryo did not damage the rest of the embryo nor hinder its further growth. In the following year they employed the technique for the benefit of several couples with a history of an X-linked condition enabling the selection of only female, and therefore unaffected embryos. Male embryos, because of the risk of their being affected, were not implanted. The technique can also prevent unnecessary abortion because for certain X-linked conditions termination of male pregnancies following sex diagnosis by amniocentesis or chorionic villus sampling results in the termination of an unaffected fetus in half the cases. Another benefit is that the results of the tests are available within a few hours which allows unaffected embryos to be implanted without freezing.

PCR has also been used by Winston, together with Robert Williamson and other collaborators, to detect the genes cystic fibrosis (CF) and Duchenne muscular dystrophy (DMD). Their targets were a stretch of DNA close to the mutation responsible for cystic fibrosis, and part of the sequence coding for dystrophin, which when mutated causes DMD. They studied unfertilized eggs: the technique has not yet been extended to single cells removed from embryos, so cannot yet be applied clinically. Using PCR to screen for specific diseases would have obvious advantages over screening for sex alone: those diseases which are not X-linked, such as CF, could be included in the screening, and for X-linked diseases, such as DMD, unaffected male embryos could be detected and implanted where previously they might have been unnecessarily discarded.

In developing these procedures, animal models proved of great value. Using biochemical detection of enzyme defects, and PCR to detect DNA defects, Marilyn Monk and her colleagues in London were able reliably to screen preimplantation embryos from mouse strains carrying genes equivalent to those responsible for the human genetic disorders Lesch-Nyhan disease and beta thalassaemia. The diagnoses were carried out *in vitro*, on cells removed at the 8-cell stage, and validated by allowing the operated embryos to develop in a surrogate mother. Monk and Holding went on to show on human material that sickle cell disease could be diagnosed by amplifying the surplus DNA discarded by the unfertilized egg into the first polar body. This approach holds considerable promise from the clinical point of view, since it does not require manipulation of the embryo.

Principles of gene therapy

Whether we are considering somatic cell gene therapy or germ-line gene therapy, there are three types of approach that might be used to overcome malfunctions at the genetic level. The most obvious version of gene therapy would be gene replacement—the replacing of mutant genes, which fail to do their job properly, with normal ones. Conditions to be treated must therefore be those caused by single defective genes. The gene must have been identified and cloned, and techniques would be required for ejecting the aberrant gene and splicing in a normal version. A second alternative is gene correction—the alteration of a malfunctioning gene by a technique such as site directed mutagenesis to put right its erroneous coded message. Although this appears at least as difficult as the replacing of a faulty gene, genetic sequences have been modified in several different types of mammalian cell. The most promising approach at the moment, however, is gene augmentation. This means introducing a fully functional gene into a cell without first removing or changing the resident, non-functional mutant gene.

Whatever the technique adopted for somatic cell gene therapy, the gene would have to be inserted into (or modified within) cells in the affected tissue. This is clearly a much simpler prospect for a tissue such as blood or bone marrow, which can be removed, treated in the laboratory, and reinjected, than for tissues such as liver or brain. Because all such approaches are still essentially experimental, diseases to be tackled by genetic modification are also likely to be very severe conditions for which there is no effective alternative treatment.

Some of the earliest theoretical targets for gene therapy were sickle cell anaemia and other haemoglobin disorders. However, work in animals has shown that conditions of this sort are far from easy to correct, largely because of the difficulty of bringing transferred genes under proper control.

Somatic cell gene therapy—the first steps

The earliest concrete moves towards somatic cell gene therapy, taken in the last two or three years, have been centred on four very different conditions. First, cells carrying the mutant gene responsible for most cases of cystic fibrosis have been corrected by insertion of the normal gene. Although accomplished in laboratory glassware rather than in patients, this achievement confirms the feasibility of overcoming genetic defects by genetic modification.

Two groups announced the breakthrough in September 1990. One team used a retrovirus to ferry the normal gene into a pancreatic cancer cell derived from a patient with CF. The gene began working, producing the protein whose absence causes the characteristic symptoms of CF. The other team attained the same objective by using a modified vaccinia virus to insert the gene into cells derived from those that line the human airways. There is still a long way to go—not least in learning how to ferry the gene into airway cells in a human subject—before these findings can be expected to help CF patients. One possibility is to introduce the gene by using as the vector an adenovirus, a type of virus that occurs naturally in the respiratory tract.

In the second advance, similar to the CF work, researchers inserted a normal gene into lymphocytes from a patient with the rare genetic disorder known as leucocyte adhesion deficiency, which leaves victims exposed to recurrent, life-threatening infections. Using a retrovirus as the vector, they introduced a normal CD18 gene to compensate for the aberrant CD18 gene that is responsible for the condition. The gene was expressed, causing the cells to behave normally. There are now hopes of transferring the gene into stem cells. This could lead to the formation of a new population of normal lymphocytes in human patients.

The third breakthrough, in 1989–90, was reported by Steven Rosenberg, W. French Anderson, and others at the National Cancer Institute and National Heart, Lung, and Blood Institute in Bethesda, USA. Their long-term aim is to optimize the treatment of certain malignant diseases by using the patients' own tumour-infiltrating lymphocytes (one type of white blood cell) together with interleukin-2. This is a natural substance which stimulates growth of the lymphocytes that attack what they recognize as foreign tissue. In their preliminary work, the researchers took lymphocytes from patients suffering from advanced melanoma and then used a virus to introduce into the nuclei of the cells a gene conferring resistance to a particular antibiotic. This enabled them to monitor the survival and behaviour of the cells when reinjected into patients. Strictly speaking, therefore, the procedure (which was successful and free of side-effects) was an exercise in gene marking rather than gene therapy. More recently, however, the same approach has been adopted to enhance the tumour-destroying capacity of lymphocytes, by giving them genes to overproduce a potent protein called tumour necrosis factor.

A fourth advance which has become the first real example of human gene therapy, is targeted against severe combined immunodeficiency disease (SCID), a rare disorder affecting about forty children world-wide each year. In nearly half of the patients studied, the gene for the enzyme adenosine deaminase is defective. The end-result of this deficiency is that the individual's immune system is severely impaired in its capacity to defend the body against invading microbes. Efforts to tackle the disease using gene therapy, devised by French Anderson and colleagues, involve taking lymphocytes from SCID patients, introducing a normal gene coding for the enzyme, and then transfusing the white cells back into the patient. The first attempt at this was carried out on a 4-year-old girl in September 1990. Within just a few months the girl's immune system was showing signs of action and in less than a year her bloodstream contained normal amounts of disease fighting white blood cells.

Cancer and gene therapy

As most human cancers are probably associated with aberrant expression of genes, cancer can be considered a genetic disease. Some research suggests that gene transfer might be used to combat malignant conditions such as retinoblastoma, which seem to follow the inactivation of a cancer suppressor gene. Other avenues of enquiry include inactivation of the oncogenes that are responsible for many cancers, and the introduction into tumour cells of genes making them uniquely sensitive to particular drugs.

The Human Genome Project (HGP)

> When finally interpreted, the genetic messages encoded within our DNA molecules will provide the ultimate answers to the chemical underpinnings of human existence. They will not only help us understand how we function as human beings, but will also explain, at the chemical level, the role of genetic factors in a multitude of diseases, such as cancer, Alzheimer's disease, and schizophrenia, that diminish the individual lives of so many people.

So wrote James Watson, co-discoverer of the DNA double helix in a recent article in the journal *Science* (Watson 1990: 44). Now director of the US National Center for Human Genome Research, Watson was commenting on the launching of a project which is being heralded as the biological equivalent of the 1960s Apollo project to put astronauts on the moon. The ultimate aim of this massive international programme is to map the positions of all of the 100,000 or so genes on the human chromosomes—and possibly eventually to determine the entire human DNA sequence of some three billion base pairs. The cost of obtaining the total sequence is estimated at $3 billion. For the more immediate purpose of initiating the mapping effort, the US government has committed over $150 million for the year 1991, while the sum of spending by European countries and the EC is nearly $20 million.

Given that the positions of only 4 per cent of human genes have so far been located, and that only a handful of the 4,000 or so recognized genetic diseases have been traced to their malfunctioning genes, the potential value of the Human Genome Project for medicine may be enormous. The research has three broad goals. Small parts of each have already been achieved, before the inception of a co-ordinated mega-project, by the sort of research described in this and earlier chapters. First, a genetic map is being constructed. This is done by recording the frequencies with which particular characteristics are co-inherited, and thus inferring the proximity of the corresponding genes on the chromosomes. A genetic map indicates the general, but not absolute, positions of the genes.

A physical map, on the other hand, shows the distances between particular landmarks in terms of the actual length of DNA. Compiling such a map is a relatively new pursuit, based on the idea of breaking up the genome into manageable pieces, identifying the fragments, and then determining how they relate to each other. There are hopes that the Human Genome Project will facilitate the production of such a map, showing major landmarks, within five years.

Sequencing is based on tried and tested methods although their speed and efficiency are being continually improved, as are methods of handling the vast amount of data generated. Some biologists, particularly in the USA, see the compiling of a complete sequence for the human genome as a holy grail. The majority view is that such an effort would not be a worthwhile use of resources. At the centre of this argument is the riddle that only about 3 per cent of the DNA in the human genome (like that in other higher animals) is devoted to genes. The rest, often described as junk, may be important over evolutionary times as a source of new genes, but is of little interest for medical or other practical reasons.

The largest fragments of DNA that can be sequenced consist of 300–500 base pairs. So even an average gene, which is 2–3 times longer than this, has to be broken down into smaller pieces. Several different restriction enzymes have to be used on any one stretch of DNA, producing overlapping sequences of base pairs that can be matched up to give the entire sequence. When a genome is chopped up into manageable chunks, those pieces are stored as a 'library'. Each fragment is inserted into a microbe and thus cloned. This is usually done using either E. coli (in which the inserted fragments, containing some 40,000 base pairs, are known as cosmids) or yeast (in which the pieces, called yeast artificial chromosomes, can be from 250,000 to a million base pairs).

Sydney Brenner has argued that as the Human Genome Project moves forward, only a few hundred bases need be sequenced at the end of each gene. Apart from indicating whether that gene has already been sequenced, this would also provide enough information to indicate the type of protein encoded by the gene. Researchers could then decide whether that gene is likely to be of any interest.

Compiling other genomes

The first complete DNA sequences ever established were those of tiny DNA viruses, which contain some 5,000 base pairs. The largest single piece of DNA yet fully sequenced is the genome of cytomegalovirus, which has about 250,000 base pairs. Several laboratories around the world are now tackling the bacterium E. coli, with about five million base pairs. In a programme initiated in January 1989 under the European Community's Biotechnology Action Programme, twenty-five laboratories in ten European countries have been sequencing the 370,000 base pairs of an entire yeast chromosome, and are now moving on to three more of yeast's complement of sixteen chromosomes. One outcome of this work should be the discovery of previously unknown genes, and thus the determination of their functions in the cell.

Another international effort, centred in Cambridge, has the goal of sequencing the 100 million base pairs in the genome of the worm Caenorhabditis elegans. This work had its origins in a project launched by Sydney Brenner in the early 1960s to compile a complete description of the genetics, molecular biology, and developmental biology of this tiny organism, which is less than a millimetre long and consists of a mere 959 cells. Although there is still some way to go, *C. elegans* is already the most completely understood of all multicellular organisms.

Research interest in the genetics of the mouse began to take off during the 1950s when increasing similarities were noticed between the genes of mice and those of humans. Indeed, in some cases, genes for human diseases were only assigned to their positions on the human chromosomes after the corresponding genes were mapped in the mouse. Gradually, a more detailed map of the mouse genome has been compiled and over 2,600 genes have now been located.

European researchers in sixteen different centres have also begun working towards a map of the pig genome, initially by seeking markers whose co-inheritance with particular genes can be monitored. There are likely to be mutual spin-offs between this work and the Human Genome Project, not least because there seem to be many parallels between the two animals. Genes that occupy adjacent positions on the human genome, for example, are likely to do so in the pig as well.

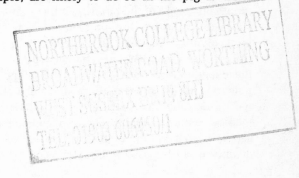

Chapter Nine

Current Laws and Guide-lines

Throughout the 1970s and 1980s there has been increasing concern with the health and environmental consequences of new technologies. This has led to new, and more rigorous, standards for the assessment of new products and processes. It has also led to calls for more public information and greater public involvement in deciding whether the possible risks arising from such products and processes are acceptable. Biotechnology regulation has been something of a test case for putting into practice some of these new approaches and principles.

The key difficulty in regulating a new technology is that the nature and scale of the hazards, if there are any, is not known. How do we solve the problem of regulating the risks of biotechnology when we do not know with any certainty what the problems may be? This chapter will examine and evaluate the experience various countries have had of regulating the potential health and environmental risks of biotechnology. It will finish by considering the regulation of certain new medical biotechnologies. Detailed consideration of a further aspect of regulation, that of patenting genetically modified organisms is discussed in Chapter 11.

The changing nature of regulation

It is only in the last twenty-five years that extensive regulation of the hazards of industrial products and processes has become commonplace in even developed countries. governments have instituted some controls in response to adverse health, safety, and, more recently, environmental effects. Legislation has been passed, based on the experience of adverse effects, requiring that the product or process attain certain standards of health, safety, and, where appropriate, efficacy and environmental protection. One example of such reactive regulation is the Medicines Act, passed in 1968 as a response to the thalidomide tragedy of 1962.

The irreversible, and potentially catastrophic, nature of our damage to the environment led some to argue that we needed a *proactive* or precautionary approach to environmental decision-making. Instead of responding to hazards once they had occurred, it was proposed that we should anticipate and control them by careful prior assessment. From the start, the proactive approach has been a major strategy in regulating biotechnology.

At first sight anticipation of risks seems far superior to the trial and error of reactive regulation, but it has serious limitations arising from the difficulty of evaluating the future consequences of a previously untried event. The nature or conditions surrounding the occurrence of the hazards we are attempting to anticipate may be unknown. Very often our understanding of hazards is most readily advanced by analysis of actual events, sometimes involving accidents.

The approach of 'sophisticated trial and error' attempts to combine the advantages of trial and error with that of anticipation. It involves use of analysis to protect against the most serious risks and advocates erring on the side of caution. Meanwhile small-scale trials are permitted and monitored so that the opportunity to learn more about the possible hazards is maximized. Risk assessment experiments are designed to test specific hypotheses about the hazards and to gather more empirical information. Even this approach suffers from the limitation that some of the most serious risks may go unrecognized.

The recombinant DNA controversy of the 1970s

When the techniques of gene splicing first emerged in 1972–3 several molecular biologists raised the question of the safety of moving DNA between distantly related species. Some believed that the natural barriers to gene transfer were there for a good reason and to transgress them might have dangerous consequences. Conjectural hazards included the accidental move-ment of cancer-inducing, pathogenic, or other deleterious genes to common micro-organisms and the subsequent infec-tion of laboratory workers, or members of the public.

In 1974 a group of eminent molecular biologists published a letter in the journals *Nature* and *Science* proposing a moratorium on certain types of recombinant DNA (rDNA) work. The voluntary adoption of that moratorium by American and European scientists has been recognized as a unique episode, a point made by the philosopher Jerome Ravetz:

It was quite unprecedented in the whole history of science for a group of scientists to call for a halt to their work, and trust to the force of consensus to ensure that colleagues in other countries did not cheat. If Leo Szilard had been successful in his efforts to get such a moratorium among the much smaller group of atomic scientists in 1938, the subsequent history of the world would have been much simpler and safer. (Ravetz 1990)

In 1975–6 the moratorium was lifted for most experiments and a set of guide-lines developed which graded the potential risks and established an appropriate level of physical contain-ment (including, for example, negative air pressure in laborat-ories, air-locks, air filters, etc.). In addition, crippled or weakened micro-organisms were developed (for example which could only survive in the presence of a rare substrate) as a form of biological containment. The aim of containment was to prevent the escape of a genetically modified organism, or components used in its manufacture (the host, vector, and so on) from the reaction vessel and from the laboratory.

The first rDNA guide-lines were very stringent but were relaxed within a few years. They continued to be relaxed so that today 90 per cent of rDNA work is subject to the minimal control of 'good laboratory practice'. The most important reason for the relaxation of the guide-lines appears to have been the emergence of a new consensus amongst molecular biologists in the latter years of the 1970s that the conjectural risks were in principle no different from those of naturally occurring pathogens. If pathogens were not employed in rDNA work it was extremely unlikely that one would be created because pathogenicity is a complex, multi-gene trait. Furthermore no cases of illness amongst laboratory workers performing rDNA work emerged, and several risk assessment experiments provided reassuring results.

The regulation of rDNA research provides a good example of the sophisticated trial and error approach: it involved treading cautiously initially, relaxing conditions as more empirical and theoretical knowledge justified this. Certainly the approach managed to secure the confidence of trade unions, industry, and the majority of scientists, at least in the European context. The downside is that the research developed very slowly at first and considerable time and money was spent by scientists and governments in assessing risks and building high containment facilities.

We would be mistaken, however, to become complacent when considering the possible risks of rDNA research, as the case described below demonstrates.

Deaths at the Pasteur Institute—a warning?

During the 1980s concern was expressed that the deaths from cancer of seven scientists from the Pasteur Institute, Paris, might be related to their involvement in rDNA research. An investigation revealed that the overall cancer rate of the Institute's workers was lower than that of a random sample (this being due to the smaller proportion of smokers at the Institute) but that there were higher rates of bone cancer in men and pancreatic cancer in women. The rates for brain tumours and leukaemia were also higher than expected, although the numbers were too small to be statistically significant. The authorities concluded that people working at the Institute *may* run a greater risk of contracting certain cancers but the investigation did not establish whether the cause was exposure to rDNA or to carcinogenic chemicals which were used in the research. Partly in response to the Pasteur Institute's report, the International Agency for Research on Cancer (IARC) has commenced a mortality study of 'biology research laboratory workers'.

Concern about working with certain types of naked DNA sequences grew when a team at Glasgow found that the DNA sequence of oncogenes could cause tumours, with or without treatment with tumour promoters, when applied directly to the broken skin of mice. Although the work did not establish a definite risk to humans there was a tightening up of the British guide-lines on work with oncogenes.

Industrial applications

Large-scale research and development and production using genetically modified micro-organisms began in earnest in the mid-1980s. Strict containment of large volumes of micro-organisms was very difficult and expensive, although it had been achieved for some time with the manufacture of vaccines from pathogenic micro-organisms. Companies using disabled strains questioned whether it was necessary to kill off micro-organisms in effluent, given that the organisms would die rapidly outside the fermenter. After all, the brewers and bakers, and even the antibiotic makers, are not required to treat effluent in such a way that all micro-organisms are killed (though they often do for commercial reasons). Another issue was the possible allergic response of factory workers to rDNA organisms, or their products. Cases of allergic reactions have been reported from a number of factories producing amino acids, single-cell protein, contraceptive hormones, and enzymes for biological washing powders.

A working group of the Organization for Economic Co-opera-

tion and Development (OECD) recommended that manufacturers should employ organisms which were intrinsically
low-risk (for example biologically crippled) wherever possible.
Such organisms could be employed under conditions of Good
Industrial Large-Scale Practice (GILSP), meaning the current
best practice in industrial biotechnology using safe micro-
organisms. Nearly all large-scale applications to date have used
the GILSP category and no adverse health or environmental
effects have been reported. Indeed there may even be greater
health and safety problems in the traditional biotechnology
industry than in the new biotechnology.

Environmental and agricultural applications

Management of risks by containment is, of course, impossible
when the intention is the deliberate release into the environment of genetically modified organisms. Risk management
must then rely to a great extent upon assessment of the adverse
effects, if any, of the organism upon its environment, an
assessment rendered extremely difficult by our lack of
knowledge and understanding of ecological systems.

Three principles for regulating releases have become widely
accepted. First, that regulations ought to be tailored to the
nature of the organism and the environment into which it is
introduced, rather than to the method (genetic modification as
against traditional mutation and selection) by which it was
produced. This point was strongly endorsed in *Introduction of
Recombinant DNA—Engineered Organisms into the Environment: Key Issues*, a report published in 1987 by a US National
Academy of Sciences committee. It follows wide acceptance of
the argument that a microbe or plant that has received a new
gene as a result of recombinant DNA work cannot be
distinguished from one that has received the same gene
through more natural processes. Secondly, that the risks of
each release should be assessed individually (case by case)
because, as yet, it is not possible to apply general principles.
Thirdly, releases should take place step by step, meaning that a

genetically modified organism should be tested first in the laboratory, then in glasshouses, then during a small field trial, followed by a larger field trial, then trials in different environments, and so on until marketing. Step-by-step development allows researchers to learn continually and make appropriate modifications to their development programme.

It is clear that the approach presently adopted corresponds closely to the sophisticated trial and error model. Risk assessment research is being performed in an attempt to understand better the possible hazards, much of it funded by governments, including European Community programmes, and by seed and agrochemical companies. There are pressures, however, for the current approach to change. On one side are some environmental activists, who have argued that no releases should be conducted until we can be confident that no environmental damage will occur (i.e. trial *without* error). On the other side are some molecular biologists and industrialists who want to move away from the relatively cautious approach. They argue that regulation of hypothetical hazards is strangling innovation because it renders research and development prohibitively costly. The problems with both of the above arguments can be inferred from the already mentioned limitations of trial and error and anticipation.

It is probable that the potential hazards of release will be most acute when genetically modified organisms are used commercially by many users (e.g. farmers). It will then be more difficult to control the use of organisms, or to monitor their effects, and there is the additional problem of interference effects between genetically modified organisms. There is no guarantee that there will not be adverse effects, but these must be put into perspective. The damage may be less than that caused by the use of alternative technologies (chemical pesticides and fertilizers). It is also worth considering that the possible ecological disruption arising through use of genetically modified organisms is unlikely to come close to the damage wreaked upon the environment by the creation of agricultural land by deforestation.

Risks from products

When genetically modified animals and plants are finally used in agriculture, food regulators will question whether the insertion of new genes has altered the food's nutritional or toxicological properties. How should consumers be informed, if at all, of the use of genetic modification in a product's manufacture? Will the genetic modification of vaccines alter their safety? Regulators, scientists, industrialists, and consumer groups are just beginning to consider such issues. The Ministry of Agriculture in the UK, for example, has recently recommended that manufacturers employ special labelling when the use of genetic modification materially alters the nature of the food.

Current controls in the European Community

There is a considerable convergence in the laws and guide-lines devised to regulate biotechnology in the industrialized countries. This is a reflection of the increasingly globalized character of economic, social, and scientific activities. The principles of regulating new technologies are established increasingly in international fora such as the OECD and the United Nations. In the case of EC countries, the establishment of harmonized regulation to complete the single market by the end of 1992 has been a major motivation behind the development of a number of Directives regulating biotechnology.

The provisions of Directives have to be translated into national laws. One Directive (90/219/EEC) regulates the contained use of genetically modified micro-organisms in laboratories and factories and requires that scientists and companies conduct a risk assessment of the proposed activity. A regulatory authority must be established in each member state, which will administer notification or authorization procedures depending on the scale and the environmental risk of the particular operation. Provision of certain information to the public is guaranteed and the authority may involve the public in its decision-making. Information must be shared between member states and countries may present objections to a particular facility or project in another country. A second Directive (90/220/EEC) regulates the deliberate release of genetically modified organisms, providing for the establishment of national regulatory authorities and similar public information requirements as the first Directive. Each individual experimental or trial release will need consent from the national authorities and a summary will be sent to the other member states for information. For marketing a product containing a genetically modified organism, all twelve national authorities will have to consent to the proposed placing upon the Community market. If there is disagreement between member states a final decision can be made by a committee of member states representatives by a qualified majority vote. Both these Directives should have been implemented into the national law of all member states by 23 October 1991.

There has been much controversy recently concerning these Directives, especially that regulating releases. Industry, and many scientists, have objected to the 'singling out' for regulatory purposes of the techniques of genetic modification in the absence of a scientific basis for so doing. It is feared that the public will assume that genetic modification is more dangerous than other techniques because it is regulated separately from them. There are, nevertheless, a number of convincing arguments for special regulation; for example, a cautious approach requires it and no existing legislation would cover certain applications. People have questioned, however, whether the Directives are sufficiently flexible to be changed as knowledge and experience accumulates.

A further Directive to protect workers from the occupational risks of using biological agents has been passed. A number of other Directives regulating biotechnology have been proposed but not as yet passed, for example one on marketing genetically modified plants and one on transporting genetically modified organisms.

United Kingdom

In the UK, health and safety aspects of work involving genetic modification are regulated by the general Health and Safety at Work etc. Act 1974, which is administered by the Health and Safety Executive (HSE). There is a legal obligation for employers to inform the HSE of genetic modification work and to conduct an appropriate risk assessment. A committee of scientific experts and representatives of trade unions, industry, and central and local government (the Advisory Committee on Genetic Modification—ACGM) gives advice to the HSE and other government departments about risk assessment of particular projects and regulation in general. The ACGM and its predecessor the Genetic Manipulation Advisory Group (GMAG), have played a key role in developing regulation in the UK, especially through their guide-lines on particular aspects of genetic modification work.

In November 1978, GMAG published a discussion paper setting out the basis of a possible new system for the categorization of genetic modification experiments in the UK. It became known as the Brenner risk assessment following its conception by Dr Sydney Brenner, Director of the MRC Laboratory of Molecular Biology in Cambridge.

The assessment is based on consideration of three factors relevant to transmission and pathogenicity of genetically modified micro-organisms:

1. *Access factor* (A): the probability that modified organisms, if they escape, will enter the human body (that is initially of the laboratory worker), that they will survive there, and that they will penetrate membranes so as to reach the tissues containing susceptible cells.
2. *Expression factor* (E): the probability that the foreign gene in the modified organism will be efficiently translated into the protein product of the gene and that the products will then be secreted from the altered organism.
3. *Damage factor* (D): the probability that the product of expression of the foreign gene will cause physiological

damage in the body of the individual to which it gains access.

The HSE and ACGM in the UK require the local safety committee to review the numerical assessment of risk based on these three factors on the scale of 1 (maximum risk) to 10^{-12} (lowest risk). The probabilities are multiplied and the final figure is used as a ranking on which to base the level of laboratory containment necessary. Approximately 95 per cent of all experiments carried out to date in the UK have been assigned to the lowest level of risk (less than 10^{-15}). If it is considered impossible to assess a particular property of the construct, it has been customary, in keeping with the general approach in the UK, to adopt a cautious approach and score a higher level of risk than may be necessary, until further information is available.

The environmental aspects of genetic modification are regulated under Part 6 of the Environmental Protection Act 1990, implemented by the Department of the Environment (DoE). Under this law, which was much influenced by the EC Directives and a report from the Royal Commission on Environmental Pollution (1989), deliberate releases of genetically modified organisms will require consent from the Secretary of state for the Environment and from the HSE, who will receive advice on a case-by-case review from the Advisory Committee on Releases to the Environment (ACRE). This committee is composed of, among others, scientific and environmental experts, industrialists, and trade unionists. Information about applications to release genetically modified organisms, as well as ACRE's advice to the Secretary of State, will be placed upon registers of information available to the public.

An important component of regulation in the UK has been its openness to outsiders. Scientists have been encouraged to issue press releases to local newspapers and to answer enquiries from members of the public. A further component of the government's approach to regulating biotechnology has been to reassure the public that the possible risks are being recognized and addressed. The HSE and DoE issued their new draft regulations for public comment in the form of a consultation paper in October 1991.

Federal Republic of Germany

There has been much interest from political parties, professional societies, local groups, and the scientific community in Germany in the debate about the possible risks and benefits of biotechnology. The Greens have traditionally taken a strong line against all uses of genetic modification, seeing it as the ultimate domination of nature. More Greens are now taking a less fundamental line, however, and seeing the benefits of some applications (for example in producing new pharmaceuticals).

There were a number of well-publicized confrontations between the Greens and the German chemical industry in the 1980s over whether to construct biotechnology plants. Most infamous was the five-year long dispute over Hoechst's plans to build a facility producing human insulin from *E. coli*. The development was continually held up by legal challenges from local groups, who claimed that the possible environmental risks were unacceptable. Several major German firms (e.g. Bayer and BASF) decided to move some of their biotechnology research, development, and production operations to the USA, partly because of the scale of the opposition. In addition to regulatory delays, some research facilities have been bombed and set alight by groups believed to be attached to the Red Army Faction.

The situation has changed by the lessening of the political influence of the German Greens and by the passing of the Genetic Engineering Act in July 1990, which has made it much more difficult for groups to oppose construction of plants in which it is planned to use genetically modified micro-organisms classified as being of no risk. Most commercial applications fall into this category and four plants using genetically modified micro-organisms have been granted licences since the law was passed. So far only one deliberate release has taken place in Germany and this evoked considerable controversy. The Contained Use Directive will be controlled in Germany at state level whilst the Deliberate Release Directive will operate through the Federal Health Ministry (Bundes-gesundheitsamt).

Other EC countries

Those EC countries with specific legislation controlling genetic modification prior to the EC Directives include Denmark (1986) and the Netherlands (1990), both of which have adopted a reasonably cautious policy. Several other EC countries have no specific regulation of genetic modification (Italy, Greece, Portugal), though this does not prevent other laws being used where applicable. Of the European countries, the largest number of releases of genetically modified organisms have taken place in France. A release committee under the auspices of the Ministry of Agriculture examines proposed releases, though the system is at present voluntary and subject to much secrecy. Scientists and companies are not encouraged to give information to the public about their experimental releases, or to liaise with local officials. Belgium is another country in which a large number of releases have taken place, including large-scale trials with the vaccinia rabies vaccine. By 23 October 1991 all the member states should have established a statutory regulatory system by implementing national laws based on the two EC Directives.

The United States

Instead of creating new laws to regulate genetic modification as in the EC, this US government is adapting existing legislation to the task. This has led to the establishment of biotechnology safety committees in various government agencies including the Environment Protection Agency, the Department of Agriculture, and the Food and Drug Administration. Some of the earliest releases of genetically modified organisms took place in the USA, sometimes leading to clashes with local and environmental groups. By the end of 1990 there had been 132 releases of genetically modified organisms in the USA, slightly more than in Europe. A complicating factor in the USA is the ability of the individual states to pass regulation to control genetic modification work in their territory and several (including New Jersey and Wisconsin) have done so.

There has been strong pressure recently from the White House's Council on Competitiveness, chaired by Vice-President Quayle, to deregulate biotechnology. According to the Council's proposals a genetically modified organism need not be subject to federal regulation unless there is substantial evidence that it presents 'unreasonable' risks. This amounts to a move away from the cautious approach presently in operation in the USA and Europe and has aroused much opposition from environmentalists, ecologists, and even from some companies.

Regulation of medical biotechnologies

The enormous advances in medical biotechnologies are raising many ethical, safety, and legal questions to which regulatory answers will have to be provided. Several governments have responded to the growing calls from scientists to conduct research on embryos by drafting legislation permitting this up to a limit of seven or fourteen days post-fertilization (France and the UK respectively) or prohibiting such research (Germany). The cloning of humans, construction of hybrid species with humans, and the modification of human germ-line cells are strictly forbidden under the UK's Human Fertilization and Embryology Act 1990. The proposed French Bioethics Law goes further in attempting to maintain the 'dignity of the individual' in the wake of rapid advances in medicine. Any research which threatens the integrity of humans or leads to eugenic practices is banned. There are attempts afoot in the Council of Europe to establish an international bioethics committee to ensure the same basic ethical rules are followed in all twenty-four member countries. The Commission of the EC established a working group on embryo research in 1990 and is intending to establish an advisory structure on ethics and biotechnology.

Possible health risks arise from the use of new biotechnologies. Yet the safety and efficacy of medical technologies, such as in vitro fertilization (IVF), are not assessed in the same rigorous way as new pharmaceuticals. According to some observers, for example, the effects of superovulating hormones on the woman's health during IVF have not been thoroughly investigated.

Somatic cell gene therapy experiments are unregulated in many countries, including the UK, although it has been suggested that they pose health risks arising from the activation of deleterious genes by retroviral vectors. In the USA the rDNA guide-lines cover gene therapy experiments and federally funded proposals must be approved by several committees of the National Institutes of Health. In 1989 the Department of Health in the UK established a committee on the ethics of gene therapy 'to draw up ethical guidance for the medical profession on treatment of genetic disorders ... by genetic modification' and to advise on particular proposals. The Committee's response was published in January 1992. In short, it gives ethical approval to somatic cell gene therapy in severely ill patients but concludes that the modification of germ cells should not yet be attempted. The government has given both organizations and individuals the opportunity to comment on the report's conclusions and recommendations before deciding what steps to take. Its final response is expected later in 1992.

Chapter Ten

The Implications of Genetic Modification in Animals, Plants, and Micro-organisms

The genetic modification of plants, animals, and micro-organisms has been one of the main areas of biotechnological research and has the potential to generate substantial benefits for human and animal welfare and for our environment. Some processes involving genetically modified organisms are already in use. For example, bacterial fermentation is already being used not just to improve the extraction of copper from mining operations, but also to clean up mine wastes and thereby to reduce toxic environmental contamination. There is, moreover, substantial scope for the use of genetically modified organisms to improve the disposal and utilization of farm animal wastes, and conceivably also to develop animals which produce less noxious wastes. The genetic modification of organisms is, however, not entirely free of risks or problems.

Potential benefits and risks

Agricultural productivity in Britain has grown rapidly and more or less continuously for approximately 250 years. Similar growth rates in agricultural productivity have been achieved in many other countries too, particularly in other parts of the industrialized world. Technological change has played a major role in raising agricultural productivity, and genetic modification has the potential to contribute to sustaining, or even accelerating, that long-term growth trend.

Despite the obvious attractions of improving the economic performance of farming and horticulture, questions have inevitably been raised about the desirability of a rapid rate of innovation in those circumstances in which we now find ourselves, namely a European agricultural regime burdened by substantial and growing surpluses of numerous agricultural commodities. It may well be that some improvements in agricultural technology are highly desirable, but it may also be necessary to give careful consideration to the selection of those innovations which should most readily be implemented.

Historical experience

International experience gained by the development and introduction of new and substantially more productive varieties of grain into developing countries, a process which has come to be known as the 'Green Revolution', can provide historical lessons which might usefully guide the new phase of scientific research and industrial innovation made possible by development of genetic modification. The social impact of the Green Revolution is itself a matter of some dispute. While it had the potential to improve the quality of life, the bulk of the evidence suggests that the impact of the introduction of new short-stemmed, high-yielding varieties of rice, wheat, and maize varied depending on the social context into which they were introduced, with the result that it was often a technical success but a social disaster. Frequently the introduction of Green Revolution varieties increased agricultural productivity and total crop yields, but also increased the total number of hungry and starving people. This paradoxical outcome was a consequence of the technical characteristics of the hybrid seeds and of the social inequalities which prevailed in the communities into which they were introduced. How did this situation come about?

Typically, Green Revolution varieties were more productive than traditional varieties, but only under a restricted set of conditions. To optimize their productivity, they generally required relatively large inputs of water, fertilizer, herbicides, and pesticides. The seeds themselves, and the irrigation and chemicals required to provide the conditions they needed, inevitably made the new varieties much more expensive than the traditional ones. As a consequence, relatively wealthy farmers increased their harvests and incomes, while the standard of living of poorer farmers declined steeply to the point where a large proportion of them lost their farms and joined the ranks of the homeless in search of an income. The only regions in which the impact of the Green Revolution was generally beneficial were those such as Kerala in Southern India and in parts of Taiwan where substantial disparities between farmers did not exist. Under those circumstances agricultural production and income levels generally grew across the board.

More recently, Green Revolution plant breeding institutes have sought to develop high-yielding crop varieties which will be less dependent upon scarce or expensive inputs, and which can produce a satisfactory crop even in suboptimal conditions. However desirable their efforts may be, there is a risk that any improvements which they create will arrive too late to enable large numbers of displaced farmers and farm workers to re-establish themselves.

It may have been difficult, or even impossible, for scientists working in the Green Revolution plant breeding laboratories during the early 1960s to foresee the eventual impact of their work. However, with the benefit of experience, it is reasonable to expect experts, who are trying to select particular genetic characteristics for plants and animals, to have careful and prior regard to the probable consequences of the application of their work beyond the laboratory. In other words, researchers have an ethical duty to consider the consequences of their work on both communities and the environment. Three examples illustrate some of the things we need to consider before altering plants in ways which on a superficial level seem to be wholly beneficial.

First, if the techniques of genetic modification are being used to develop crop strains which can tolerate or even thrive in the presence of herbicides, one might also consider the differential impact within the farming community of the introduction of such varieties, as well as their propensity to increase the use of synthetic herbicides. (Considerations of that nature are relevant not merely to the eventual conclusions of governmental regulators and commercial farmers, but could also be relevant determinants of the prior research and development objectives of genetic scientists.)

The second example comes from research intended to genetically modify plants capable of fixing their own nitrogen. The successful completion of this research would be broadly welcomed, partly because it would substantially reduce expenditure on fertilizers and dependence on the energy-intensive methods of their production, and partly because it would reduce the environmentally undesirable contamination of ground water from the application of nitrogenous fertilizers. Questions have been asked, however, about the risk of possibly transferring the plants' ability to fix atmospheric nitrogen to other species which are already weeds, or which could consequently become weeds. Similarly, there could be the risk of herbicide or pesticide resistance in crops being transferred to weeds. Although such questions should not prevent research on genetic modification of plants going ahead, it is important for those working in this area to ask themselves whether or not these concerns are realistic. If we are to benefit from the genetic modification of food crops, great care will need to be taken to try to foresee possible pitfalls, and to take steps to avoid them, rather than to proceed as if all the difficulties which need to be overcome are purely technical.

Finally, while the potential benefits of genetic modification to agriculture in the developing world may be at least as great as those promised to the industrialized countries, problems may also arise. If it were, for example, possible to use genetic modification synthetically to manufacture delicious flavourings such as those of coffee and vanilla, without having to extract them from tropical agriculture, then the livelihood of some tropical farmers might be threatened. The benefits of reducing domestic consumer prices therefore may need to be weighed against the possible economic consequences to those countries which depend on the revenue from the export of such crops for their economic development.

Genetic modification of animals

While the genetic modification of plants is generally widely accepted, within carefully controlled limits, the modification of animals is not so readily condoned by the public as is evident from the vociferous campaign activities of the animal rights and animal welfare lobbies. The former believe that animals should never be used by society for anything. They also argue that while people may do what they like with their own species as far as genetic modification is concerned, it is quite unacceptable hubris for people to decide to manipulate other species. The latter, in contrast, condemn some but not all uses of animals by society and campaign to improve the welfare of those animals through, for example, more humane methods of rearing, transport, and slaughter.

Many of the arguments against genetic modification in animals still centre on such issues as whether or not people are justified in exploiting animals as food or in causing them pain to satisfy purely human needs. Consensus is unlikely to be reached on these matters but most people would agree that animals should not suffer needlessly nor be killed without good cause. As long as the extent of animal genetic modification lies within these boundaries therefore people will be more likely to support the development and use of genetically modified animals. The use of transgenic animals, for example, to produce pharmaceutical products for the treatment of disease such as haemophilia is generally met with greater approval because the suffering to the animals concerned is minimal while the benefit to haemophiliacs is substantial.

Some uses of transgenic animals, however, have come under greater criticism, particularly those which are used as models of disease. The oncomouse, for example, caused particular concern among those interested in animal welfare because it was deliberately developed with an increased susceptibility towards cancer. The mouse caused still further controversy when its developers applied for and were subsequently granted a patent in the United states in 1988. Although transgenic animals may be valuable for research into the molecular biology and treatment of diseases their suffering, arguably, may not justify the research. Before accepting the use of genetically modified animals in medical research the benefits accrued to our understanding of disease must therefore significantly outweigh the possible suffering of the animals concerned, as required by the Animals (Scientific Procedures) Act 1986. Some critics, however, would raise the objection that as it is people who make decisions regarding animal experimentation there is likely to be an inbuilt bias which will tend to underestimate an animal's suffering.

Turning to agriculture, as mentioned previously pedigree livestock can now be cloned to produce lots of genetically identical animals with improved milk- or meat-yielding capabilities. In addition to the general arguments about the ethics of breeding animals for food, new arguments specifically against cloning have been raised which focus on the issue of genetic diversity.

The maintainance of genetic diversity

A great deal of concern has understandably been expressed about the risks of a possible reduction in, or loss of, genetic diversity amongst both plants and animals if genetically modified varieties were to come to dominate commercial agriculture and horticulture. That concern is based, partly, on the assumption that genetic diversity helps species to survive the hazards of a changing environment, such as climate and soil conditions and, in addition, inhibits the spread of pathogens: parasites, bacteria, viruses, or moulds which affect some varieties of a species may leave others untroubled. Therefore if too many of our agricultural eggs are confined in too few genetic baskets, then we might risk losing the whole lot.

Moreover, because the environmental and pathogenic conditions in which our agriculture is operating are constantly changing, plant and animal scientists may be required to tackle challenges in the future which at present are impossible to predict. Therefore, the greater the diversity of plants and animals with which they can work, the more readily they will be able to meet these challenges as they are encountered. For this reason we need to retain some stocks of thriving plants and animals as potential breeding stock, even if they are not being used immediately or directly for agricultural or commercial purposes. Although that argument is broadly acknowledged, there is a debate about how, and by whom, those genetic stocks should be held. During recent years in Britain, steps have been taken to divest the public sector of their plant and animal gene banks, by selling them into the private sector and generally to large agrochemical companies. It remains to be seen what impact those new arrangements have on science and agriculture, but it is possible that commercial firms might decide that some activities which government scientists were perfectly willing to engage in, such as sharing their stocks, will become subjected to commercial constraints to the detriment of the public interest.

The environmental release of genetically modified organisms

One of the main focuses of the complex debate about the social and environmental consequences of the application of biotechnology is the deliberate release of genetically modified organisms into the environment. There has, in particular, been a great deal of controversy over this topic in the USA, Germany, and Denmark, but the corresponding debate in the UK has, so far, been relatively muted and far less comprehensive because opposition has been virtually absent. Nonetheless, public concern about the release of such organisms into the general environment is more extensive than any anxiety about the modification of organisms which remain confined within the laboratory. However, the benefits of genetic modification can frequently be obtained only by the broader dissemination of the organisms concerned.

The potential benefits from the environmental introduction of helpful and useful organisms need to be weighed against the possibility of unwanted adverse consequences which may arise from their release. A hazard may be posed because the genetically modified organisms will, for the most part, only be useful if they can survive and multiply. Occasionally some benefits might accrue from the use of disabled organisms that are able to survive out of the laboratory for only a short time, for example baculoviruses against the pine beauty moth, but more commonly that would be impractical. Problems might arise, however, if genetically modified organisms either transferred their genetic novelties to other species in which their expression would be unhelpful or positively harmful either to those species or to their environment, or if the novel organisms mutated, survived, thrived, and multiplied and then transferred their genes to other organisms.

There is no agreement within the scientific community about how plausible or probable such adverse developments may be. Some scientists and industrialists draw attention to, and comfort from, the fact that little or no demonstrable harm has resulted from any of the experimental releases which have occurred thus far.

When the 'ice minus' bacteria were released into commercially cultivated crops, some scientists were anxious that the novel organisms might compete not just with bacteria against which they were targeted, but that they might also provide

frost protection to other plant species, which might consequently become more robust than is desirable.

Typically, scientists have defended their experiments and
the commercial application of their results by arguing that the
introduction of genetically modified organisms is less likely to
cause problems than the innumerable unintended random
mutations which have occurred over evolutionary time. They
argue, moreover, that because the novel genetic modifications
have been carefully selected and modified they are likely to be
less hazardous than either natural evolutionary processes or
traditional methods of breeding plants and animals. One
response to that line of argument has been to insist that when a
natural mutation occurs, it will typically occur in isolation,
while the environmental release of genetically modified
organisms will involve the simultaneous release of very large
populations of thriving and robust novelties, and therefore any
adverse or undesirable interactions are more probable.

The fact that a genetically modified organism has been
modified to a relatively high level of precision does not
necessarily guarantee that its environmental impact can be
reliably predicted. Scientists still know too little about the
relationship between, for example, genetics and morphology,
let alone between genetics and ecology, to be able to predict
confidently how the release of a large population of genetically
modified organisms will interact with all the other species that
inhabit the environment into which they are being introduced.
While the probability of an adverse transfer of genetic material
may be very low, the consequences of such transfers might be
very serious.

Criteria for judging the environmental release of genetically modified organisms

Among the issues currently being debated in professional
circles are the considerations and criteria according to which

the environmental release of genetically modified organisms should be judged acceptable. Inevitably, some participants in the debates would like to see those judgements based variously on a broader or narrower range of considerations. Rather than concentrating their energies on that debate, industrial managers often argue that what is more important is that the criteria should be clear and precise rather than vague and amorphous.

The criteria which official advisory committees adopt will almost certainly evolve, but in any case it is desirable that, prior to its release, a genetically modified organism should have been developed in a step-by-step fashion so that data is available from studies in contained facilities such as laboratories, growth rooms, glasshouses, etc. before small-scale release and subsequent large-scale releases are carried out. Information should be available not only with respect to the interaction of the genetically modified organism with target species (in the case of a vaccine or pesticide) but with other species in the environment. An effort will need to be made to forecast its environmental trajectory, to improve the researchers' ability to select which tests to conduct, and which genes to engineer. The ways in which a genetically modified population of novel organisms can reproduce will obviously need to be a key consideration, as will be the size of the population to be released, and the variability in the conditions in which they might be used.

It is very difficult to imagine being able to reverse any genetic changes which might occur as the result of the environmental release of genetically modified organisms and it would at least therefore be desirable if the novel organisms carried some recognizable and distinctive characteristic. This might be conceived as a sort of genetic bar-code which all carriers of the modified genes might bear, and that should facilitate keeping track of their location, impact, and evolution. Such an arrangement might be beneficial not just to public and environmental health but also to research in environmental science.

The regulation of the genetic modification of animals and novel foods

The Animals (Scientific Procedures) Act 1986 is one of the UK's laws regulating biotechnology in living vertebrates. The Act imposes strict controls on the use of living animals in research and requires each programme of work to be justified in advance. Before a transgenic animal can be produced a project licence must be granted by the Home Office. In assessing whether or not to grant a licence, the Secretary of state has to weigh the likely adverse effects on the animals against the benefit likely to accrue from the research. The term 'adverse effects' is all embracing, covering pain, suffering, and distress or lasting harm. Similar considerations have to be taken into account before an animal is released from control of the 1986 Act. This weighing of 'cost' is a significant factor in protecting and maintaining animal welfare. The Advisory Committee on Genetic Modification too has produced guidelines for researchers on safety, animal welfare, and environmental issues that might be raised by the generation of transgenic animals.

The Advisory Committee on Novel Foods and Processes, which is an independent body of experts, advises Ministers of Health and Agriculture on any matters relating to the manufacture of novel foods or foods produced by novel processes. The Committee considers all foods, including those produced by technology involving genetic modification, which might bring about significant toxicological or nutritional changes in people. During 1989 the Committee assessed its first genetically modified product—a strain of bakers' yeast which produces the enzymes responsible for dough fermentation at a faster rate than other yeasts. Having evaluated the potential hazard to consumers of the yeast and of foods in which it is present, the Committee came to the conclusion that it posed no threat to human health and safety. The ACGM and the Food Advisory Committee (FAC) also approved the yeast and in March 1990 the government cleared its use by bakers.

The decision has caused some public concern because the FAC did not consider it necessary to attach special labelling requirements to the sale of products containing the genetically modified yeast, the reason being that the origin of the genetic material introduced was a strain of the same species of yeast. However, in the interests of openness it is important that consumers are informed when foods contain genetically modified ingredients. Labelling requirements ought therefore to be introduced.

Chapter Eleven

The Patenting of Genetically Modified Organisms

Of all the topics on the policy agenda in relation to genetic modification, the topic of patents for genetically modified organisms has perhaps received most attention, and the reason why can readily be appreciated: the patenting of life-forms is breaking completely new ground, giving rise to thorny questions about whether life can, or should, be 'owned'. From the point of view of commercial and industrial enterprises these questions are considered academic and they are more immediately concerned with the practicalities of gaining a financial reward for their creativity. Industrial biotechnological research is expensive and becoming increasingly so. Of the total expenditure which a company might devote to the innovation of a new product, a typical pattern includes spending some 20 per cent of the total budget on research, while the remaining 80 per cent is absorbed by development costs. One can readily understand therefore why a science-based industrial company might conclude that they should either obtain a rate of return on their investments in genetic modification commensurate with those available in all other technological sectors, or else stay out of the genetic modification industry. The industrialist's perspective is, however, not the only point of view.

Objections to patenting animals and plants

Animal rights groups, some environmentalists, and many religious groups have expressed doubts about the morality of permitting patents for plants and animals. They argue that companies do not have the right to hold a monopoly on modified organisms, a situation essentially the same as 'owning' life. The World Council of Churches was concerned particularly with this idea. Granting a patent on living organisms, it argued, removes the distinction between living and non-living matter and undermines the unique status that life is accorded.

Those involved in farming have also long been opposed to any regime which would grant the same kind of patents rights to animal and plant breeders as are available to the manufacturers of items of inanimate technology, because such an arrangement would deprive farmers of the rights to the offspring of their own stock. The very viability of agriculture has, since the neolithic revolution, depended on farmers using some of last season's crop as seed for the next. If plants and animals were patentable, then the company in possession of the patent would be entitled to consequent rights on all the offspring of the plants and animals, and would be entitled to prevent, or charge for, the use of seeds saved from one year's crop.

The European Patent Convention (EPC), which was established in 1973, recognized the force of those arguments, and established a regime under which patents could be granted on micro-organisms and microbiological processes, but which explicitly precluded patents on all plant and animal varieties. According to the philosophy underlying the EPC, plants and animals must be treated differently from inanimate objects. The biotechnology industry, however, is calling for a reform of the patenting system which would allow plants and animals to be treated, for legal purposes, just like inanimate technologies. This is being strongly opposed by some animal welfare organizations which have been calling on the government to encourage the European Community to redraft the Treaty of Rome so that animals are classified as 'sentient beings' and not 'agricultural products or goods'.

Patents and the law

In 1980, the US Supreme Court decided that under US law genetically modified organisms could be patented. Its decision meant, in effect, that any living species could be patented; not just microbiological organisms, but plants and animals too, provided they were the product of manufacture. During the 1980s, patents for several genetically modified plants were granted in the USA, and in 1988 the oncomouse was the first animal ever to be patented.

In Europe, patenting laws are currently not so liberal. The current legal position in France is closer to that which the biotechnology industry would like to see throughout the European Community and which is envisaged under a new draft EC Directive on the patenting of 'biotechnological inventions'. For example, a farmer in Burgundy has already been prosecuted for sowing seeds from the previous year's harvest. Some manufacturers have gone so far as to suggest that rather than sell their patented seeds, they may opt for contract arrangements with the farmers under which they would only lease the stock, but not sell it, thereby retaining a far greater degree of control than would otherwise be possible and than they have enjoyed hitherto.

The European Commission published the draft Directive in response to calls from industrial interests, and because it was concerned to ensure that European industry did not find itself at a competitive disadvantage when compared with, for example, American and Japanese companies. If accepted, the Directive would go a long way to dismantling the current legal barriers to the patenting of biological entities. There are problems, however, because the draft Directive is inconsistent with the EPC, and because it is strongly opposed by some agricultural, environmental, and animal rights groups. The

EPC says that 'essentially biological processes cannot be patented'. Consequently a legalistic and linguistic debate has arisen about the precise scope of terms such as 'biological' and 'microbiological'.

The EPC specifically states that 'varieties' of plants and animals may not be patented. In the mid-1980s the Munich-based European Patent Office (EPO) set a precedent by deciding that a single plant fell outside the scope of the expression 'plant variety', and was therefore not precluded from being patented under the provisions of the Convention. In taking that decision the boundary between what is and is not patentable was shifted in a more liberal direction, one which was welcomed by the biotechnology industry, but one which correspondingly alarmed some agricultural and environmental groups. In October 1991, the EPO extended its criteria of patentability still further and granted its first patent on an animal, the oncomouse, bringing Europe in line with the USA.

In 1989 the EPO examiners had rejected an application from Harvard University to patent its genetically modified oncomouse in Europe. The reason which the EPO gave for their rejection of the application was because they did not have sufficient information with which to decide whether or not the oncomice constituted a genuinely distinct variety of the species. Following an appeal, the issue again came under review, and the recent judgement has accepted that oncomouse is not an animal variety but the result of a microbiological process.

This decision alone, however, does not satisfy the necessary criteria for the granting of a patent. In the EPC there is a further important provision which requires not merely utility and originality on the part of every patentable invention, but also that their use must not be prejudicial to 'public morality' and 'public order'. This meant deciding whether animal suffering or environmental threat caused by the invention outweighed its benefits for medicine. The appeals board decided that the role of the oncomouse in advancing cancer research and treatment was of such importance to the welfare of mankind that it far outweighed its drawbacks and consequently did not constitute a public threat. On the basis of this decision therefore a patent was granted. The EPO has stressed that the decision to patent the oncomouse will not lead automatically to the granting of patents on all transgenic animals. Further applications will all be assessed individually and the examiners may reach different conclusions. However, opponents to the patenting of animals argue that now a precedent has been set the EPO may find it increasingly difficult to deny applicants a patent on their transgenic inventions.

The oncomouse, and the award of a patent for it, are not without their critics. A normal healthy mouse might reasonably expect to live for approximately eighteen months. The genetic modification of oncomice entails that within six months of birth almost every mouse develops fatal tumours. Animal welfare groups have characterized it as having been 'designed and bred to suffer', and argue therefore that this violates the standard of 'public morality'. The pattern of tumour development characteristic of the oncomouse has, moreover, no obvious parallel in the growth and development of human tumours, and therefore some scientists have questioned the utility of the oncomouse, and consequently raised, at least implicitly, questions about its suitability for a patent.

Plant breeders' rights

The ratification in 1961 of the International Convention for the Protection of New Varieties of Plants (the UPOV convention), established a formal system of Plant Breeders' Rights (PBR). PBR was built upon long-standing, but relatively informal, historical arrangements and is still in force. PBR provides some genuine, though strictly limited, protection to the commercial interest of plant breeders. Historically, the decision as to whether or not a novel plant for which registration was being claimed amounted to a genuinely novel variety was made by professional plant breeders acting collectively.

Increasingly, however, such decisions are being argued over, not just by scientists but by lawyers, and decisions are more and more being taken out of the hands of the scientists.

Under the current PBR system farmers are formally entitled to exercise what is called 'the farmers' privilege' which allows farmers to re-sow all and any of their own seeds. Under PBR, moreover, there is a system supposed to guarantee free access to, and exchange of, genetic materials between research scientists. If the proposed EC Patents Directive were implemented as drafted, it would deprive farmers of some of their historical rights, and almost certainly restrict the free exchange of breeding material. If this were to happen, it is likely that it would increase the competitive advantage of large farmers over small farmers, and would disadvantage small agricultural breeders by comparison with the large agrochemical and biotechnology companies.

Criticisms of the EC draft patenting Directive

The European Commission's draft Directive on the patenting of biotechnological inventions has itself been interpreted in several conflicting ways. It formally states that naturally occurring plant and animal varieties should not be patented. It proposes, however, that plant and animal components or products may be patented just so long as they are available as a result of some patentable human processing intervention. On some interpretations, the level of intervention required might be as slight as a process of extraction or purification, and if that interpretation is correct the Directive would in effect permit the patenting of plants and animals, despite explicit statements to the contrary. The interpretation preferred by the British government, and their position on this delicate policy point, remains to be clarified, and no plans have been announced to introduce similar legislative changes in the UK.

The formal rationale offered by the Commission is that the traditional arrangements embodied in the EPC were founded on an outdated set of technological possibilities, and on a distinction between what is biological and what is micro-biological. The Commission argues, as do some but by no means all biologists, that the development of molecular genetics dissolves the apparent contrast between what is microbiological and what might perhaps have been called macrobiological. Even if it were correct that the supposedly clear contrast has subsequently been shown to have been a spurious distinction, the question remains whether the macro should be assimilated to the micro or vice versa. In other words, there is a choice to be made whether patent rights should be extended to the entire living world, or whether patents should be disallowed even for micro-organisms. Either the arguments in favour of the farmers' privilege and plant breeders' rights were sound in 1961 and they should not be weakened by innovations in genetic modification, or those arguments should not even have been accepted under histori-cal conditions.

Given that patenting of the products of genetic modification is now lawful in the USA, the European Commission can reasonably argue that they have to consider the need to ensure that the European biotechnology industry is not systematically disadvantaged in world trade, but due regard should also be given to the interests of farmers and environmental interests too, as well as 'public morality' and 'public order'. There may be excellent reasons for trying to achieve a harmonized international patent regime, but the European position does not have to be directly based on the American model. It is just as much in the American's interest to compromise on these matters with their trading partners as it is for the Europeans to gain access to American markets and technologies.

One specific criticism of the draft Directive has been that it amounts to a total break with the traditional policy that naturally occurring plants and animals may not be patented. According to a common interpretation of the Directive, it implies that an organism can be counted as 'novel', and consequently be eligible for a patent, merely if it has not previously been recorded in the scientific literature, even if it has been present for millions of years. Many developing countries fear that large agrochemical companies will collect samples of their plants and animals, and patent the important genes, without the benefits of those patents accruing to the countries from which they were taken, or to the farmers who have conserved them through history. Consequently, some developing countries have instituted bans on the export of their flora and fauna.

While the EPC includes provisions which exclude the granting of patents to products or processes which offend 'public morality' and 'public order', no such corresponding provisions have been included in the draft Directive. Since animal welfare groups oppose the patenting of animals such as the oncomouse, they interpret the absence of any morality provision in the Directive as an undesirable omission, and a distinct weakening of the level of protection currently offered to laboratory animals under the European Community's Directive for the protection of animals used for experimental and other scientific purposes.

Adverse comment has also been focused on the provisions within the draft Directive concerning the burden of proof in the event of a dispute. Under the current regime, the burden of proof in a case alleging a possible infringement of a patent lies with the plaintiff. The individual or company bringing the complaint has to produce evidence that their patent has been infringed. The proposed Directive would, however, shift the burden of proof onto the defendant. It would require, for example, that farmers alleged to have kept and sowed some seeds from a previous genetically modified harvest, or bred from patented animals, would have to prove that they had not actually done so. It is difficult to imagine precisely how a farmer could meet such a challenge. Possibly the farmer would need to produce a complete and exhaustive set of receipted invoices to have any defence against such allegations. In addition, the proposal to reverse the burden of proof would erode the strong presumption, in English common law, of innocence until guilt is proved. If those provisions of the

Directive were incorporated into European Community legislation then a situation would develop in which the use of genetically modified strains of plants and animals might be confined to large commercial farms, and the balance of comparative advantage would shift even further against small farmers.

The problems of international differences between patenting laws

Patenting in general, and the possibility of patenting the products and processes of genetic modification in particular, raises a complex set of legal, ethical, and practical problems. To register a patent, it is necessary to provide sufficient information to enable anyone else to copy the process or product, although they may have to pay for that privilege. In the case of a genetic modification patent, it may not be sufficient to follow normal procedures with the patenting of inanimate inventions and merely to describe the process in words and pictures. It may be necessary actually to deposit a sample of the relevant organism with a patent office so that other people can draw on their genetically modified stock.

In the hope of ensuring that penicillin would be generally available, and that its availability would not be restricted by commercial considerations, Alexander Fleming and his colleagues refused to apply for a patent on penicillin. That strategy, however, backfired because instead the United states Department of Agriculture (USDA) obtained a patent on penicillin, and subsequently British researchers and pharmaceutical companies had to pay the USDA for making and using it. This problem highlights one of the dilemmas confronting the policy debate. The European Community may decline to adopt the proposed Directive on patenting the products of biotechnology, and stick with the current provisions of the EPC, but that by itself will not prevent companies from obtaining patent protection in, for example, the United states. To encourage reform in the EC, industrial companies engaged in biotechnology and especially genetic modification argue that if the level of patent protection within the EC is weaker than that afforded to them in other markets they will simply relocate their laboratories and factories in more favourable and welcoming climates.

The threats of commercialism to scientific collaboration

The accelerating transformation of scientific and technological research and knowledge into marketable commodities, not just in genetic modification but in other fields too, is undermining many of the traditional and desirable aspects of scientific work and collaboration. For example, the dispute between researchers at the University of California at Los Angeles and the Hoffman La Roche Corporation concerning commercial rights in relation to interferons, inhibited the traditional and informal free exchange of scientific information and research materials. In the long run these changes may have, and might even already be having, adverse effects on the protection and promotion of public health. For example, it has been argued that the dispute which arose between the Pasteur Institute and the US National Cancer Institute over the commercial rights to a test for antibodies to HIV delayed the introduction of tests for this pathogen, with the consequence that numerous blood samples remained unscreened, and the virus may therefore have infected many more people than might otherwise have been the case.

Patenting the human genome

Exceptional problems are expected to arise in connection with possible applications for patents arising from research on the Human Genome Project. These matters will be reviewed in greater detail in Chapter 14, but in this context it is important to appreciate that the results of research to sequence and map human genes cannot comfortably be accommodated within either current or proposed patenting legislation. The foremost dilemma raised is whether human DNA should be patented at all. A gene sequence, after all, is a description of an already existing 'product'—it is not an invention. A further dilemma arises because if a scientist were to attempt to patent a sequence as soon as it is discovered, then it would almost certainly not be possible to satisfy the condition requiring utility of the entity to be patented, but by the time that condition was satisfied, it would fail the standard of novelty. In the UK, this paradox has not yet been satisfactorily resolved and the applicability of patenting to genes, particularly to human genes, remains to be tested in the courts. One proposal, however, has suggested that it might be possible and desirable to introduce a period of grace during which the disclosure of technical information might occur without prejudicing any subsequent application for a patent, and correspondingly to increase the length of any patent which may subsequently be granted. Such a proposal has already been established in the USA, which allows a period of grace of one year, and also in Japan which grants a period of six months.

Proposals for resolving the patenting issue

It is generally recognized that the current EPC is inconsistent with some of the key aspects of the proposed patenting Directive, and neither the EPC nor the draft Directive are consistent with legislation in the USA. In these circumstances it may be appropriate to have a broader and fuller debate on all the industrial, social, and ethical issues which have been raised, before establishing a new patenting regime which may not receive the desired level of public and industrial support.

One possible approach might be to allow the patenting of a carefully defined subset of non-human organisms, on the condition that patenting of human genes was explicitly ruled out. An acceptable regime might also allow farmers to breed from their stock without having to pay a licence fee to the patent holder. Companies developing genetically modified seed might, however, respond by deliberately choosing only to market first generation hybrids, the seeds from which are less productive, in order to try to ensure that one year's crop could not be used as next year's seeds.

As was suggested in an article in *New Scientist* (Watts 1991), one compromise might be to amend the draft Directive to allow patents only on the first generation of a new plant or animal, with the proviso that breeders and farmers may freely use all genes at any time to improve species by traditional breeding techniques. While that idea may be plausible and attractive, it does not deal with the possibility of inserting some human genes into an agricultural animal. There is nothing approaching a consensus on the issue of whether or not that should be patentable.

In the context of this discussion of patents on plants and animals, it may also be appropriate to refer to the *Moore* case which occurred in the USA, where a team of doctors used some cells removed from a patient during therapeutic surgery, and then bred those cells and obtained a patent on them. The courts subsequently decided that the person from whom they had come had few rights over them. One focus of the debate concerning those events was on the question of whether the patient would have given informed consent to the removal of some of his tissue if he had known that it might be used in that way. The university in which the cell breeding occurred, and which obtained the patent, responded by arguing that the potential utility of the patient's cell line emerged only after the tissue had been taken from him, and the informed consent which he gave was quite sufficient at the time of surgery and for the purposes for which it was given. In the UK, the MRC took steps to create a fetal tissue bank of material obtained from abortions and miscarriages, and to control the use of such tissues and to reduce the risk of controversy, but questions of ownership have not been addressed adequately.

Pressure is mounting from the biotechnology industry for legal resolution of all the difficult issues raised in this chapter. However, care must be taken not to bow to this pressure until

all the questions have been addressed thoroughly in broad and
public debate with representations from all the different
interest groups.

Chapter Twelve

The Implications of the Application of Genetic Modification to Pharmaceutical Products

Many potential benefits from the application of genetic modification to the production of drugs and chemicals have been forecast. As mentioned in earlier chapters, animals, plants, and micro-organisms already have been genetically modified to produce hormones and proteins which are useful for treating a number of diseases. New safer and more effective vaccines are also being developed to prevent debilitating diseases such as influenza or hepatitis B. By the end of the century it is expected that the production of most drugs will involve biotechnology to some extent.

Genetic modification, furthermore, may be valuable for reducing the cost and improving the efficacy and purity of some of the pharmaceutical ingredients with which we are already familiar. In so far as it achieves this end, development should be encouraged, but it does not mean that a drug which is already permitted should be manufactured by a novel genetically modified process and accepted without any further question. There may be, for example, a potential risk that the genetic modification process could introduce contamination with microbial pathogens which traditional methods of manufacture avoided.

Human insulin versus pig insulin

A controversy has arisen over the use of synthetic human insulin for treating diabetics. Traditionally, insulin extracted from the pancreas of pigs or sheep was used to treat sufferers of this disease. However, since 1982 human insulin manufactured using the techniques of the new genetics has increasingly taken over from animal insulin. On switching to the new human product many diabetics (10 per cent of UK sufferers) have complained that they have suffered an alarming increase in hypoglycaemic (low blood sugar) attacks due to a loss of warning symptoms. Whether there is a link between human insulin and the frequency of attacks is currently under fierce debate with studies finding conflicting results. The issue is not resolved but the experience demonstrates the need for caution in introducing new pharmaceutical products for the treatment of disease, whether manufactured using genetic techniques or otherwise.

The opportunity costs of genetic modification

While the application of the techniques of genetic modification to the production of chemical and pharmaceutical products attracts more public support and fewer criticisms than most other parts of genetic modification, some research scientists who are not working with genetic modification have expressed some concern that there may be adverse effects if the funding for non-genetics-related medical and biological research is consequently curtailed. But there is, so far, little evidence that problems of that sort are occurring.

The 'fourth hurdle': the need for genetic modification

The only remaining distinctive social and ethical issue concerning this field of genetic modification to have risen on to the public agenda has become embodied within the debate over the so-called 'fourth hurdle'. The word 'hurdle' is used to refer to the criteria which have to be satisfied if a pharmaceutical product is to be granted a product licence, and allowed on to the market. The three accepted, and relatively unproblematic, hurdles concern the safety, efficacy, and quality (i.e. the purity) of a drug product. The proposed and highly controversial fourth hurdle would involve judgements of the social need for, and impact of, a new technological innovation.

In relation to the genetically modified hormone bovine somatotropin (BST), which the biotechnology industry wishes to market to the dairy industry to help raise milk yields, an argument has arisen to the effect that over and above the three normal criteria which are routinely applied to all drug products, this fourth hurdle should be added to cover the social and economic aspect of the use of that compound, and others in a similar category. In that context a dispute has ensued as to precisely which types of products and processes might fall within the newly designated regulatory category.

There are several versions of the fourth hurdle proposal. The most explicit proposal, which is embodied in a draft Regulation from the European Commission's Agricultural Directorate is intended to apply to applications for permission to market animal pharmaceutical products if those compounds are intended for administration to healthy animals or for yield-promoting purposes, as distinct from those intended for therapeutic, prophylactic, or clinical purposes. The Commission's proposed regulation calls for a fourth hurdle review under the following headings: socio-economic impact (including on individual farms, and structural and regional impacts), environmental impacts, effects on quality of agricultural products, and ethical considerations, including animal welfare, possible methods of control, and market impact.

The anxiety aroused by, and the opposition to, this proposal comes primarily from the biotechnology and pharmaceutical industries. They are apparently fearful that if such a fourth criterion were invoked in relation to non-therapeutic uses of genetically modified products, its application would rapidly be extended to cover some or all products of conventional (non-genetically modified) technologies and also to animal and human pharmaceutical products with prophylactic or therapeutic uses. They see it, therefore, as potentially the thin end of an extremely long and ever-thickening wedge.

Two distinct strategies have been invoked by those opposing the introduction of any such fourth hurdle. The first response is to argue that while social and ethical judgements need to be made, they should be made in the market-place and not by government regulators. On this argument, if customers find the application or consequences of a technology unacceptable then they will not buy it, and it will fail in the market-place. The second approach is to argue that official regulatory judgements concerning the approval or otherwise of a technological innovation should rely on, and only upon, objective scientific facts, and not be undermined by, or muddled up with, subjective social and political considerations.

Shortcomings in those two responses have, however, been pointed out. In the case of BST, the market-place could only function as a means to convey a signal of public disapproval if, at the very least, all milk supplies were labelled to indicate whether or not BST had been used in their production, but that is not what is being officially proposed. While labelling would be a necessary condition for the expressions of social judgements in the market-place, it would not necessarily be sufficient. An adequate level of public understanding would also be required, as well as the availability of alternative supplies, in order to protect the public interest.

The first argument might also be vitiated by the fact that the particular interests of each individual farmer are not necessarily consistent with the collective interests of the agricultural sector as a whole. If individual dairy farmers can raise their productivity by 20 per cent then they will have a comparative market advantage, but if all dairy farmers adopt the same technology then, without any growth in the total market for dairy products, an average of 20 per cent of the dairy farms will be driven out of business. Alternatively, the size of herds may diminish. It may, in the medium to long term, be desirable for agricultural productivity to rise and for the number of people engaged in farming in the EC to decline, but the scale of social disruption which a very rapid shake out in dairy farming would cause might be difficult to manage.

If the EC did not have a responsibility to manage agricultural change then there would be less pressure on EC regulators to consider the social and economic consequences of the introduction of a compound like BST, but given that the Common Agricultural Policy is in operation it would be irresponsible for one section of the European Commission to take a decision which could cause major problems for another section without ensuring that both sets of considerations were taken into account. Genetically manufactured BST is claimed by its makers to be capable of raising the yield of dairy cows by approximately 20 per cent. If a new product were to be developed that promised to raise productivity by 80 per cent rather than 20 per cent, there would be no argument but that its potential social and economic impact would need to be taken into account by the regulatory process. The formal and explicit introduction of a fourth hurdle is therefore seen by some as an innovation in practice rather than principle.

A similar impression is also sometimes conveyed by the second strategy and by the debate concerning the desirability of restricting regulatory criteria to purely scientific and objective considerations. There is extensive literature which develops and illustrates the argument that judgements about the safety of agrochemical and other potential technological risks are never a purely scientific matter, and possibly never could be. The fact that the scientific community's knowledge and understanding of biology, toxicology, and ecology is uncertain and incomplete means that it is not, in general, possible for even the experts to know whether or not some compound can safely be used. In conditions of uncertainty, even the best informed experts have to make judgements as to whether or not a compound is probably acceptably safe in the light of what they know about both the risks and benefits of the intended or probable use. Social judgements about the utility of the product often, therefore, enter into the regulatory policy-making process, even constituted as it is with three rather than four hurdles. It is, perhaps, rare for policy-makers to acknowledge that fact, but then it is generally easier to defend a decision which appears to have been reached on the basis of purely scientific considerations than one which is explicitly social, political, or ethical.

One response to arguments on those lines is to say that if social and ethical considerations are difficult or impossible to avoid, then it is better that they should be acknowledged and openly described, debated, and justified than concealed or left implicit. Some government expert advisers have suggested that a fourth hurdle should be formally established to consider social needs and social consequences because if it is going to happen it should happen openly, and by reference to clearly specified, and preferably agreed, criteria. It might have the advantage, moreover, that it might then be easier to conduct a risk assessment exercise which is, or is then seen to be, socially and ethically neutral.

The strongest opposition to the introduction of a fourth hurdle, or any explicit social impact assessment, comes from some sections of the veterinary and the pharmaceutical industries. Their most forceful argument is that if such an extra requirement were to be introduced in the EC, while absent from corresponding decisions in other parts of the world, it would weaken the competitive position of European firms in world trade, and could be a cause of friction in the current Uruguay Round of negotiations for a General Agreement on Tariffs and Trade (GATT). Those who articulate the case for a fourth hurdle generally acknowledge the desirability of not leaving European industry at a competitive disadvantage but counter it by insisting that it is desirable to protect people from the adverse social effects of technological change in all countries and not merely within the European Community.

Chapter Thirteen

The Implications of the Application of Genetic Modification to People

The scope of this discussion

The previous chapter outlined some of the ways in which genetic modification might usefully and beneficially be applied to the production of new pharmaceutical products. We also considered how it might be used to develop novel ways of manufacturing drugs which are already in use. In this chapter the discussion will be confined to the direct relevance of genetic research and technology to human genes, focusing in particular on the social and ethical implications of current techniques and those which may be developed in the short and medium term.

At this relatively early stage in the development of applied genetics it is too early to be certain precisely how extensive its benefits may become. While great prospective benefits for medical science have been claimed by some protagonists, others have argued that genetic modification may have a great deal to offer to medical science but may be of less practical value to patient care. Although it might be tempting to do so, medical research policy-makers cannot adopt the passive approach of just waiting to see how extensive the practical benefits of genetic modification to patient care might be; they need to decide how best to deploy their limited resources.

Such a decision clearly cannot be made without an examination of the social and ethical implications of the techniques.

What is gene therapy?

As we have seen, genetic modification is already playing an important role in the production of drugs and chemicals for treating various human disorders. Furthermore, research into rare hereditary diseases is illuminating our understanding of more common diseases, particularly cancers and coronary heart disease. Diagnostic techniques have also been developed which can detect diseases in the fetus and so give parents the choice of whether or not to terminate a pregnancy. However, probably the most controversial potential application of genetic modification in humans is gene therapy.

Gene therapy is the genetic modification of cells of a patient in order to cure or treat diseases. The term 'gene therapy' is sometimes loosely used to describe the process by which one human trait might be swapped for a more 'desirable' one merely according to preference. This is not the way in which we will use the term. In our opinion, genetic modification should only be used to treat serious genetic disease. The possibility that some day parents may be able to 'order' children with particular characteristics such as ability to do mathematics is not only abhorrent but also unlikely ever to be achieved.

The ethical implications of gene therapy are profound and have been the subject of intensive debate for many years. The issues vary, however, according to the type of therapy. The issues raised by somatic cell gene therapy are very different from and much less complex than those raised by germ-line gene therapy.

Before looking at each in turn, it is worth considering the scope of gene therapy. Disorders caused by a defect in a single gene (**monogenic** diseases) are obvious targets for gene therapy. So far about 4,000 monogenic diseases have been identified. While most of these diseases are individually very rare, each having a frequency of only one in several thousand births or even tens of thousand births, together they affect roughly 1–2 per cent of all live-born babies. The total number of people with monogenic disorders who could potentially benefit from gene therapy is therefore quite significant.

Recent research has demonstrated that gene therapy, in the future, may also play an important role in the management of a wide range of human diseases which have a polygenic basis and which are influenced furthermore by environmental factors. Such **multifactorial** disorders include the most common and serious chronic diseases such as heart disease, cancer, and diabetes. Various approaches to treatment of these diseases using gene therapy have been under investigation, particularly with regard to cancer. For example, anti-cancer genes have been inserted into tumour cells to bring about tumour regression. Similarly, tumour infiltrating lymphocytes have been modified to increase their capacity to destroy tumours. Although such therapeutic approaches are still experimental they have shown promising results in volunteer cancer patients.

Somatic cell gene therapy

government, religious, medical, and other bodies have each addressed the ethics of somatic cell gene therapy and have all reached a similar conclusion: because genetic modification of the somatic cells affects only the individual concerned, the therapy, in principle, is no different from other routine and widely accepted therapies such as organ transplantation. As such it raises no new ethical issues but, as with any other new innovative therapies, ethical considerations regarding the testing of these therapies need to be addressed.

There must, for example, be extensive preliminary research to assess both the potential benefits and risks of the experimental treatment. To be acceptable for testing on people, the benefits of the treatment must clearly outweigh the risks. The severity of the disease will also be an important factor in judging whether the risks justify the tests. For a relatively mild affliction, one would be cautious about testing a new therapy that might have unforeseen side-effects because these might be more severe than the suffering caused by the disease itself. On the other hand, a patient with a severe or life-threatening disease is likely to be more willing to try out a new treatment, whatever the risks, because he or she would have less to lose, particularly if no other treatments have been effective. People with life-threatening diseases should not be given experimental treatments if an established one is known already to be curative.

While the immediate benefits of successful somatic cell gene therapy may be obvious, the long-term effects of the therapy may be less easy to predict. It is possible, for example, that an error in inserting new genes into a cell may transform that cell into a cancerous one, with the cancer only appearing in years to come. It is important therefore that in the excitement of developing new treatments the possible long-term health hazards of tampering with somatic cells should not be overlooked. Nevertheless, it should also be recognized that people may choose to accept the long-term risks of a treatment if it enables them to attain better health in the short term. Radiotherapy, for example, is widely accepted although it is known that it may cause cancer later in life.

Germ-line gene therapy

While somatic cell gene therapy has been judged to be ethically acceptable, germ-line gene therapy, which involves manipulating genes in the reproductive cells, presents more difficult ethical questions. This is because the effects of the modification do not die with the individual but are handed down to all future generations, thus breaking completely new therapeutic and ethical ground. At present, for a number of reasons there is a general consensus that germ-line gene therapy is unacceptable.

First, the long-term consequences of germ-line gene therapy

are currently impossible to fathom. Our knowledge of disease genes and why some persist in the population at greater frequencies than others is still too limited for us to be confident that efforts to eradicate these genes will be of long-lasting benefit to future generations. A classic example of a disease gene with an unusually high frequency in some populations is the gene for sickle cell anaemia. This gene is particularly prevalent in tropical Africa and the Mediterranean. It is now known that the gene protects carriers (i.e. those who have one disease gene and one normal gene) from malaria and as a result they have a survival advantage over both the individuals who have two normal genes and those who have two disease genes—the former being more susceptible to malaria and the latter suffering from a fatal disease. Because of this advantage, carriers are more likely to survive to have children and the disease gene will be passed onto future generations thereby maintaining it in the population.

If, without this knowledge, we had attempted through germ-line gene therapy to eradicate the sickle cell gene we would have also eradicated all the benefits that the gene confers. One might argue that these benefits are irrelevant to the large number of carriers among the black population in North America, where the mosquitoes are not malarial, and that germ-line gene therapy therefore might be justified. However, as we shall see, this argument can be countered by the fact that there are other means, less radical than germ-line gene therapy, by which individuals can be prevented from inheriting sickle cell disease. Furthermore, statistics are now showing that the incidence of the gene in the US is declining naturally because the advantage conferred to carriers no longer exists.

This example illustrates how genes which cause harm in certain environments may have an evolutionary advantage in other environments. Given this, until we have a fuller understanding of the relationship between diseases and gene action, it would be unwise to attempt to eradicate certain disease genes and thereby risk losing a gene with potential, but as yet undiscovered, value.

The second argument against germ-line gene therapy focuses on the inheritance of errors. If during the process of germ cell modification a serious error should occur by, for example, inserting a gene in the middle of another gene and disrupting its expression, this error would be handed down to all the descendants. Because the modification occurs on a microscopic scale such an error could go unnoticed and a subsequent embryo be allowed to develop. The error may not even manifest itself during the life of that person, if it is a recessive mutation, but only appear years hence as a homozygous trait in the descendants. By that time the possibility of correcting the mutation may be long past and the affected individuals and society will be required to live with the consequences. Until gene therapy can be shown to be absolutely accurate in inserting and targeting new genes, the potential hazards of genetic modification in germ cells are too grave to permit its use.

Yet another objection to germ-line gene therapy concerns the ethics of research on embryos. At present, most methods for carrying out germ-line gene therapy would require manipulating an embryo only a few days old. After modification the cells would continue to divide and, with differentiation, some would eventually become germ cells which carry the altered genotype. Research on embryos gives rise to highly emotional debate as the moral status of the early human embryo remains disputed. Consensus is unlikely ever to be reached on this particular issue as each camp—the 'pro-life' and pro-research lobbies—remain steadfast in their arguments. Despite the opposition of pro-life campaigners, legislation has nevertheless been recently introduced in the UK, under the Human Fertilization and Embryology Act 1990, which allows research on embryos up to 14 days but prohibits alteration of the genetic structure of an embryo (which would include germ-line gene therapy). Human cloning and the creation of hybrid species is also prohibited by law.

These are some of the more theoretical objections to germ-line gene therapy but there is also a very good, practical reason for opposing it. It is unnecessary. Simpler techniques can be used to prevent a disease-causing gene from being inherited, that is by preimplantation diagnosis. As already discussed this involves testing embryos for certain diseases and only selecting the healthy ones for implantation. This involves no direct tampering with an embryo's genes and so avoids the risk of genetic mutations caused by gene insertion.

There will be a few couples, however, who will not be able to benefit from preimplantation diagnosis—those who never can have a winning combination of their genes. Such a situation will arise, for example, if two people with a recessive disease, such as cystic fibrosis, decide they want children. Their children will all be affected because each parent has no normal alleles to pass on to them. It is debatable whether germ-line gene therapy, if possible, should be allowed for this minority of couples. Because the risks to future children at present are so great and the expertise still so undeveloped it is unlikely, at least in the immediate future, that germ-line gene therapy will be justified in these situations. Instead it might be considered more appropriate to offer other possibilities to these couples, such as sperm donation, backed up by all the necessary supportive counselling.

Before any genetic therapies might be considered appropriate it would be necessary to identify which people carry which genes, and this brings us to the topic of genetic screening.

Genetic screening: benefits and difficulties

Genetic screening, or the scrutiny of the genes of sections of the human population, has been taking place in a limited way for many years. For example, since the 1950s most babies born in the UK, and in many other countries too, have had their blood tested to establish whether or not they have inherited from their parents the genetic defect responsible for phenylketonuria (PKU). Children with PKU are unable to metabolize phenylalanine properly and produce a toxic molecule instead that damages the child's developing nervous system. If detected early enough the devastating effects of the disease—severe mental retardation and behavioural disorders—can be prevented by giving the baby a carefully managed diet very low in the amino acid phenylalanine. More recently it has become possible to test at various stages of pregnancy for the presence or absence of the genetic conditions responsible, for example, for Tay-Sachs disease, Huntington's disease, Duchenne muscular dystrophy, and cystic fibrosis.

The ethics of genetic screening have provoked a particularly vigorous debate within the genetic modification literature. For some enthusiasts for genetic screening, it promises a healthier, happier, and safer future, while for its critics it is unnecessary, undesirable, and pointlessly extravagant. Neither of these extremes is supportable—genetic screening can play a valuable role in promoting public health, but controls and guide-lines are required to ensure that it is not subject to abuse and that it is carried out in such a way as to optimize the balance of benefits against risks.

The consequences of genetic screening

The possible consequences of genetic screening programmes fall into two broad categories, the social consequences and the consequences for the gene pool (the total genetic information in a population). There are two schools of thought regarding the latter. Some believe that by identifying defective genes and those individuals who carry them, the frequency with which those genes occur will rapidly decline as they are, in effect, bred out of the population. Others have predicted precisely the opposite outcome, pointing out that somatic cell gene therapy and improved treatments will make it easier for people with genetic diseases to survive to have children, where previously they would have died. The effect of this therefore would be the preservation of, or even increase in, deleterious genes in the population. It should also be borne in mind that disease genes will also be maintained in the population, regardless of screening programmes, by spontaneous mutation and by carriers of a genetic disease.

The latter scenario—the preservation of bad genes in the gene pool—should not be used as an argument against adopting screening programmes since evidence suggests that it is unlikely to have a major impact on the numbers of disease genes. More genetic counselling, carrier screening, and prenatal diagnosis may be required in the short term, since there will be an increased number of carriers, but in the long term it is hoped that treatments or even cures will be developed for more genetic diseases.

The social consequences of genetic screening are far-reaching and may include stigmatization of individuals, coercion, or invasions of privacy. It is these potential problems, as well as the potential benefits offered by genetic screening, which we will be considering in the remainder of this chapter.

A gap between diagnosis and treatment

One argument which has been deployed by those who urge caution on genetic screening concerns what is often referred to as the 'gap' between diagnostic and therapeutic techniques. There is a risk that the techniques to locate and identify the presence of problematic genes are developing far more rapidly than corresponding therapeutic abilities. It may shortly be possible to provide precise diagnoses of many conditions for which no treatment is available or is likely to become readily available.

Some commentators believe that this position has already been reached. There is no treatment for Huntington's disease, for example, and there is plenty of evidence to indicate that the delay which typically occurs between developing a diagnostic technique and finding a remedy is growing. They have argued, therefore, that diagnostic information concerning genetic disorders for which no treatment or remedy is yet available should be regarded quite differently from diagnoses for conditions which can effectively and safely be treated. A careful consideration of the relationship between diagnosis and treatment should influence decisions about which screening tests to conduct, and which areas of research and development should be given priority. It would seem prudent to close the gap between treatments and diagnoses, rather than allow diagnostic abilities to run too far ahead of available treatments.

Carrier screening

Many of the common genetic diseases are recessive, that is a child would have to inherit a copy of the disease gene from both parents to be affected by the disease. People who have one copy of a recessive gene are called 'carriers' and are healthy. A programme designed to detect these people is hence called carrier screening. Carriers have a limited choice of ways to avoid having affected children: they can marry someone who is not a carrier; they can elect not to have children, or they can have pre-natal diagnosis and abort affected fetuses. For some diseases preimplantation diagnosis is also an option.

Carrier screening programmes for several genetic diseases have had mixed success. A programme in the USA to screen black people for the sickle cell trait is often cited as an example of how not to go about a screening programme.

The US experience

During the 1970s, approximately a dozen American states passed laws requiring that black people submit to genetic testing for the sickle cell trait. The screening programmes tended to target black school children or black couples applying for marriage licences. The laws disregarded the need for genetic counselling services and for protecting the confidentiality of the test results. In addition they paid little attention to the problem of the inadvertent discovery of non-paternity and to other sensitive issues.

The programme was so ill-conceived that carriers of the trait were often left with the impression that they had the disease. Parents whose children had been screened confused the trait with the disease and over-protected their children unnecessarily. Some people with the trait also faced stigmatization, being considered unsuitable for marriage or employment. Most importantly, because the focus was on a minority, racially oppressed group, the black population felt that the screening was merely a devious way to discourage black people from having children. Subsequently, the US federal government intervened by offering funds to such screening programmes, but only if they provided counselling and respected privacy and the right of individuals to choose whether to have the test or not. The damage, however, had already been done.

The Tay-Sachs screening experience—how it should be done

A contrasting illustration is provided by the programme, established in the early 1970s, to screen Ashkenazic Jews for the gene involved in Tay-Sachs disease (a devastating, recessive disease that affects the brain early in childhood, bringing death between the ages of 2 and 4). This programme has been both a technical and a social success. Approximately 25,000 Ashkenazic Jews are being tested annually in the USA, and the incidence of Tay-Sachs has been reduced by 90 per cent when compared to the period before such screening was introduced. The difference between this programme and the sickle cell programme is that the initiative came from within the Jewish community and was combined with sophisticated genetic counselling and public education.

The problem of the reliability of the genetic tests

Genetic screening programmes need to take into account problems concerning the reliability of some of the tests intended to detect the presence or absence of specific genes.

Ideally screening tests would always be entirely precise and definitive, but we are some distance from reaching that position. On occasion, currently available methods of testing produce either false positives or false negatives; that is to say they mistakenly suggest that some individuals carry genetic defects from which they are actually free, and perhaps more seriously they fail to detect some genetic problems which they were intended to locate. The kinds of problems which can occur can be illustrated by reference to the example of cystic fibrosis. The tests which are currently available can identify about 84 per cent of people carrying genes for CF. But at this level of detection, a comprehensive screening programme would identify only 71 per cent of all couples at risk of having a baby with CF, with the remaining 29 per cent slipping through the net.

Given that such a test does not identify 100 per cent of all carriers, some commentators have argued that the use of such tests can do more harm than good, because they may unnecessarily frighten some people while offering unjustified reassurance to others. However, such an argument fails to take into account the benefits of the test to the 71 per cent of couples at risk who will be identified and whose needs should also be considered. Furthermore, the concerns expressed against screening could largely be overcome by effective genetic counselling.

Genetic counsellors need to be sensitive to a wide range of social, cultural, and ethical considerations, as well as being scientifically well informed. Some commentators have even argued that before laboratories are allowed to conduct genetic screening tests they should be required to obtain a licence which would certify both their technical reliability and their proper observance of acceptable standards of ethical conduct.

The lessons learned

Clearly, before carrier screening tests can generally be recommended considerable thought needs to be given to a wide range of issues concerning the reliability and predictive power of the tests, the pre- and post-test procedures, the interpretation of the results, and the overriding social consequences of screening a population. However reliable a test is, a carrier screening programme will fail if the population is not reassured of its potential value. Therefore, the role of policy-makers, doctors, teachers, etc. is to inform society of the reasons for screening for carriers of disease, taking into account and being particularly sensitive to racial differences in disease incidence to avoid accusations of discrimination. In addition, before and after testing, supportive counselling must be provided to explain in greater detail the purpose of the test and the meaning and implications of the test results. Such counselling is essential for helping individuals and couples to understand their options and exercise them rationally. All participation in the screening programe must be voluntary and the decision of an individual not to be tested respected. A person, in addition, must give his valid consent prior to testing and the test result must subsequently be kept confidential. Carrier screening is of no obvious benefit to children and should not be carried out until they are of an age to understand the meaning of the test and give their valid consent. Only when these requirements are fully implemented will the benefits of carrier screening programmes outweigh the risks.

Pre-natal diagnosis

It is now possible to test fetuses for a growing number of genetic diseases using techniques described earlier. There are several options open to couples known to be at risk of having a child affected with a genetic disorder. They may decide not to have their fetus tested and have the baby regardless. Alternatively they may choose to have the test and on the basis of the result decide whether to seek a termination of pregnancy or not.

Genetic counselling is an essential part of the decision making process. It helps couples to understand the implications of the disease and the nature of its inheritance. Its purpose is to help the couple, non-directively, to make a decision which they feel to be right. Whatever they decide in the end to do, their decision must be respected. Genetic counsellors, doctors, and society in general therefore must be sensitive to a couple's religious, moral, or cultural beliefs, and try to be non-judgemental.

For which diseases should pre-natal diagnosis be offered and on what basis do couples decide to accept testing? The severity of the disease is likely to be a major criterion on which such decisions are based. At each end of the continuum of disease severity will be those diseases which people would tend to agree either do or do not justify termination of pregnancy. For example, terminations for lethal disorders such as Tay-Sachs disease or Duchenne muscular dystrophy are considered acceptable by most people, while terminations for cleft palate are unlikely to be accepted. Most diseases, however, fall between the two extremes. Cystic fibrosis is, for example, very unpleasant, inflicting suffering and premature death on the affected individual and causing stress and anxiety for the families. For many couples a termination for this disease would seem completely justified. Other couples, in contrast, might argue that with recent advances in medical treatment sufferers from cystic fibrosis now live longer and fuller lives and they may instead elect not to have pre-natal diagnosis. Decisions whether to accept pre-natal diagnosis may also be affected by factors such as age of onset. Many might question whether, for example, a termination is justifiable for a disease which does not manifest itself until a person is middle aged.

Criteria other than disease severity will be important in decisions concerning pre-natal diagnosis. Such criteria include the predictive value of the test, the likelihood that a child will be born with the genetic disease, and the availability of treatments for an affected child. In addition, social, moral, religious, cultural factors, and family considerations will play an important role in couples' choices. They may believe that they are not financially equipped to offer a secure life to a severely disabled child or that it would not be fair on their other children if one sibling required intensive care and attention. Their decision may also be influenced by the experiences of already having one disabled child in the family. Alternatively, a couple may simply feel it is wrong to have a termination of pregnancy regardless of the severity of the genetic disorder. As well as the clinical factors which must be satisfied before a test is introduced, these other issues must therefore be taken into account.

It is clear that the reasons why couples might choose or refuse pre-natal diagnosis for genetic disease will depend on many different factors. Decisions regarding the introduction of pre-natal screening services are therefore not only the province of those who develop and fund the tests. The debate on which services to make available should also involve policy-makers, professional bodies, patients' groups, prospective parents, and parents of children with genetic diseases to ensure that the interests of all parties are represented. It is not appropriate to pre-empt such debate by making definitive statements in this book about which diseases do or do not justify pre-natal screening services. However, we would argue that preimplantation diagnosis or pre-natal testing and subsequent termination should not be allowed for morally frivolous reasons such as for traits which have no disease association but which may not be considered 'desirable'.

Sex selection

Recently, debate has also focused on whether or not couples should be allowed to choose the sex of their baby. Sex selection is generally accepted for those at risk of having a baby with a serious sex-linked disease but its acceptability on non-medical grounds has been questioned in many quarters. In December 1991, the first centre in the UK to offer couples just such a choice opened amid a flurry of controversy. The technique does not require genetic modification but simply involves attempting to separate female X-sperm from male Y-sperm and inseminating the woman with sperm of the chosen type. The technique is reported to have an 80–85 per cent success rate for boys and a 67–70 per cent success rate for girls, although these results have not yet been confirmed in randomized clinical trials. Such success rates must be viewed against the natural 50 per cent chance of success.

Proponents of the technique expect couples who already have a number of children of one sex to be most interested in seeking the treatment. It may also seem an attractive option for people in cultural groups in which one sex has a higher status than another. But for many people the idea is simply distasteful, reducing children to the ultimate consumer product. Doctors argue moreover that it is unwise to use an unvalidated medical technique, carrying possible dangers, merely for social reasons. There are further concerns that it will lead to an increased demand for abortion because couples who find out that their fetus is of the 'wrong' sex may wish to terminate the pregnancy and try again.

Currently there is no legislation governing sex selection. As the technique usually involves artificial insemination by husband or partner, it lies outside the jurisdiction of the Human Fertilization and Embryology Authority, which licenses and oversees only those insemination centres carrying out treatments involving donated sperm. As a result, anyone wishing to establish a sex selection clinic may currently do so without regulatory control.

We consider it unacceptable to terminate a pregnancy for the sole reason that the sex of the fetus is not the one of choice. Furthermore, we would advise doctors against becoming involved in sex selection in the absence of medical need.

Testing before the onset of symptoms

A further type of screening requiring consideration is the screening of individuals for genetic disease prior to their becoming ill. The ethical problems can be best illustrated using two different examples—one involving the screening of adults at risk of Huntington's disease, the other involving screening of all new-born boys for Duchenne muscular dystrophy (DMD).

Tests have now been developed that can detect whether an individual carries the Huntington's gene or not. This is a dominant disorder—if a person inherits only one copy of the Huntington's gene he or she will develop the disease later in life. What is the value of being tested for the gene? Not knowing whether one has the gene or not may subject a person to an appalling waiting game. Every lapse of memory or clumsy movement may heighten that person's fears that he has the disease even if he does not. A person will also wonder how to plan for the future; whether to pursue a certain career or whether to have children, for example. These concerns can be settled more easily by having the test. Those who discover that they are almost certainly free of the disease will be able to plan for a 'normal' life with tremendous relief, while those with the disease gene will have their worst fears confirmed. Although such news will be shattering it should make it easier for the person to plan the future around the knowledge and to encourage him or her to continue life as fully as possible. Should, however, the patient decide not to have the test, that wish must be respected as participation in these tests must be voluntary.

If the test result is positive, accepting the diagnosis naturally will not be easy and post-test counselling has a very important role to play in helping people come to terms with the information and what it signifies. As important as post-test counselling, however, is pre-test counselling. As a candidate must give his or her valid consent prior to testing, a counsellor will need to assess a person's suitability for testing and also explain and make sure the person understands what is at stake and the choices he or she faces. Once reassured of this, given that the patient still wishes to have the test, testing can take place.

While some might question whether we should test for diseases for which there is no cure, others might argue that if individuals choose to have a test and their judgement is well informed then it should not be denied them. Although the results may not be reassuring the knowledge may still be of enormous value to those people.

Allowing the testing of children may be less easy to accept. In the case of PKU the benefit to the child is obvious as the effects of the disease can be avoided through appropriate diet. However, routine testing of all new-born boys for a disease such as Duchenne muscular dystrophy for which there is no cure raises questions. At present, only pilot studies have been carried out as to the feasibility of such a programme and there is still debate as to whether such screening should be established nationally.

There are several advantages to early screening of boys for DMD; first, early diagnosis warns parents of the risk of recurrence in subsequent children and enables them to take preventive measures if they wish. In addition, potential carriers in the family can be informed of the risks. Secondly, doctors sometimes fail to recognize the early symptoms of DMD, causing a delay in diagnosis and anxiety for parents as they seek to find out what is wrong with their child. A test would pre-empt this. Finally, the knowledge would enable parents to prepare themselves for the tasks ahead; for example, the changes in the home that will be necessary to accommodate a wheelchair.

Despite the advantages there are, however, significant disadvantages. Parents are told that their son will develop a fatal condition for which there is no cure years before the first symptoms appear. The stresses imposed by this knowledge could be profound and family relationships may be put under strain. Furthermore, the test is not always able to distinguish between DMD, which manifests itself within the first few years of life, and Becker muscular dystrophy which is a milder form of the disease with symptoms generally first appearing when boys are in their teens. Boys with DMD tend to die before 20 years of age while boys with the Becker type live much longer. This raises the question of whether parents should be subjected to the uncertainty of not knowing how severely their son will be affected. Also, if symptoms are delayed, indicating Becker form of the disease, as they grow older boys will develop an understanding of what is in store for them. This may be hard for them to accept and had they had the choice they might not have wished to know. It is difficult to decide, in this case, whether the advantages of testing outweigh the disadvantages and justify screening of new-born boys for DMD.

Confidentiality and use of genetic information by third parties

In general, and in line with all precedents in medical ethics, genetic information about an individual should be deemed to be confidential, unless disclosure to third parties has been specifically authorized by the person to whom the information relates. There are a few exceptions to the rule, such as if the law requires it or where there is an overriding public interest such as might occur in a serious criminal investigation, but generally there will be few circumstances where the release of genetic information on an individual without his or her consent is justified.

The intention of the screening initiatives discussed so far is solely to help individuals or couples make decisions about their own or their future children's lives. Screening is carried out at their request and the information gained is for use by them alone. However, information learned about one family member in relation to a genetic disease may have profound implications for other family members. How should the sharing of genetic information be handled in these cases? Currently the main reason why couples or individuals seek genetic testing is because there is a known history of the disease in the family. Family members will be aware to some extent of what this means and are likely to understand the importance of sharing information or participating in family screening for the detection of genetic markers. However, such co-operation cannot be assumed, especially with distant relations, and careful counselling may be required to inform family members of the importance of their co-operation. If a relative should refuse to be involved, health professionals must respect this.

Where there has been no previous family history, the discovery that a person is a carrier of a genetic disease will be unexpected. Other family members may benefit from this knowledge and genetic counsellors should again stress the importance of conveying the information to relatives. If the individual refuses, then any breach of confidentiality without consent would have to be justified on the basis of the severity of the disorder and implications for other family members.

Genetic screening for employment and insurance purposes also raises a host of questions regarding the use of genetic information by third parties. Such screening is quite different from the screening programmes described above. In these situations screening occurs at the request of the company not the individual, although with his consent. Results are forwarded to the company for its use in assessing fitness for employment or insurance and not for the clinical care of the individual. There is clear potential for misuse of information.

Genetic screening in the workplace

A survey conducted in the USA by the Office of Technology Assessment in 1982 revealed that six major American corporations were already using genetic tests to identify employees susceptible to adverse reactions from toxic substances in the workplace. Another fifty-nine companies said they were considering adopting such a practice within five years. Competitive pressure could well lead to widespread introduction of such practices.

If carried out with the best intentions, the genetic screening of employees for susceptibility to workplace hazards, such as poisonous chemicals or air pollutants, can have benefits for all concerned. For this to be the case, the screening needs to be optional and should be offered purely to inform current or prospective employees about the health risks they may run if they are employed in particular types of work. Having been found to have an increased susceptibility to certain occupational illnesses the choice whether to accept the risk should then be left to that individual. If the risk is great one would generally expect an employee to seek work elsewhere as few people will voluntarily choose to risk becoming ill. As a result, the person would obviously benefit by maintaining his health and the company would benefit because its costs due to occupational disease would be reduced. However, if the individual should choose to accept the risk, perhaps because the chances of other employment were remote, then the company should honour that decision and accept the consequences just as the employee would need to do.

This is an ideal situation and there is growing concern that genetic screening may be carried out by employers in order to exclude people from employment who are shown to be genetically susceptible to occupational diseases. The reasons for doing so are clear—the costs to companies of hiring people who may become ill are considerable. There will be a loss in productivity due to absenteeism, workers will require sick pay, and temporary workers will need to be hired. Another reason, sometimes cited, is that it is a cheaper alternative than cleaning up the workplace. These reasons all disregard the interests of workers and such screening therefore should not be condoned.

There is a further concern that because particular genes often occur in greater or lesser frequencies in certain racial or ethnic groups the testing for these genes will lead to the exclusion of a disproportionate number of workers of a particular racial or ethnic origin from certain industries. Accusations of discrimination will be an obvious response and employers will have to be particularly careful to demonstrate that they are exercising equal opportunities policies.

Another type of worker screening which has aroused criticism is the testing for genetic susceptibility to the major killer diseases such as cancer and heart disease, or other common problems such as mental illness. Such testing could potentially affect all workers and not just those employed in certain hazardous industries. It would therefore be particularly invidious if it became widespread. An individual tested as being susceptible to any of the above diseases may find himself or herself excluded from a whole number of jobs as employers turn him or her down as an economic risk. The result could be the formation of an underclass of workers who are either considered unemployable or unsuitable for high-ranking, responsible jobs which require a significant amount of investment in training and experience by the employers. While this may not be a problem in the immediate future, policymakers cannot ignore the risk. They must be proactive in preventing the injustices and abuse that may arise from such screening programmes.

Whatever the motives for screening employees for disease susceptibility, at present there are still many problems regarding the interpretation of results which should encourage caution over using genetic screening as a means to judging the suitability of employees for certain work. The mere presence of a 'bad' gene does not necessarily mean that a person will be more susceptible to certain workplace hazards and more likely to become ill. There is no indication, for example, that carriers of the sickle cell gene or the cystic fibrosis gene are any more disadvantaged in the workplace than a person with two normal genes. To deny a person a job, therefore, merely on the basis that he is a heterozygote for a disease gene would be completely unjustified unless there is overwhelming evidence to show that a single copy of the gene really does increase a person's risk of occupational illnesses. In addition to this, even if an increased risk of occupational illness has been associated with a particular gene, that risk may be negligible compared with the greater risks faced by all workers, regardless of their genotypes, in a given workplace. For example, the risk of an accident from using dangerous equipment in a factory is likely to be far higher than the risk of getting a certain occupational disorder which has a very low incidence (say 1 in 5,000 workers), even in genetically predisposed people. Employers, therefore, instead of making spurious judgements on the genetic suitability of workers should more readily focus their efforts on reducing the greater risks to all workers in the workplace.

Genetic information in the hands of employers who may not be sufficiently well informed to judge the significance of the information may have serious repercussions for the work-force. The use of genetic screening in the workplace therefore should move forward only very slowly and should only be adopted as it is proved that certain genotypes really do predispose individuals to some occupational illnesses. Participation in screening must be optional and the results should not be used to exclude individuals from employment but to inform them of the hazards and to allow them to make their own decisions. All genetic information about a person must be safeguarded. As genetic abnormalities are unmasked and our understanding of the relationship between genes and disease processes grows the potential for abuse will increase and guide-lines or legislation may be required to bring appropriate control to this area.

Genetic monitoring tests

The aim of genetic monitoring tests, in contrast to the screening tests described above, is not to identify individual predispositions to occupational hazards, but to detect possible genetic damage to all workers as a result of working with ionizing radiation or dangerous substances such as carcinogenic chemicals. These tests are commendable as they draw attention to the dangers of a workplace and highlight the need for action to protect the health of the whole work-force. Genetic monitoring tests ought therefore to be encouraged.

Genetic screening and insurance

Insurance companies are increasingly considering using genetic tests to assess the risk of potential policy-holders and the level of premiums they should pay on the basis of that risk. In their opinion, genetic test results are essentially no different from the other medical information insurance companies use in underwriting health insurance. Similar to current practice, those people who are found to be a low genetic risk would be required to pay only low premiums whereas those who have a high genetic risk would be required to pay higher ones or be refused insurance altogether. However, as mentioned above there are problems with the interpretation of test results which might lead to unjustified discrimination against people seeking policies: for example, there are instances of people with the gene for phenylketonuria being denied health insurance. As this disorder can be treated simply and successfully in early childhood the risk to an insurance company of expensive claims from a policy-holder with the disorder is minimal. Furthermore, an individual with a genetic predisposition to the major killer diseases such as cancer or heart disease is not inevitably destined to become ill with that disease. Other important factors, such as diet, exercise, and smoking, play an important role in the development of these diseases. Therefore to deny a person insurance or to ask for a very high premium merely on the basis of a positive genetic test result without taking other factors into account would also be unjust.

Insurance companies use a further argument to justify genetic testing. If an individual knows that he has a high genetic risk of disease that person is more likely to want to take out insurance to protect himself and his family. On the other hand, a person who finds himself at a low risk of genetic disease will think it less important to be insured. The inevitable result, the industry argues, will be an inundation of insurance applications from people with susceptibility to ill health. If an insurance company is not allowed to find out potential clients' genetic risks for itself it will be impossible for it to assess the appropriate premiums, with the risk of substantial costs being incurred. Therefore in order to protect its interests it will need to charge higher premiums for everyone, regardless of the genetic risks.

The current practice of insurance companies is to ask prospective clients whether they have information about any problem which is likely to affect their health. This being the case, anybody who had been given a positive result in a genetic screening test would be duty bound to disclose this information or risk any subsequent claim being denied. We do not feel, however, that insurance companies should be able to oblige people to have screening tests as a condition of health insurance. One might argue therefore that it would be better for people to pay higher premiums than to submit them to finding things out about themselves which they might not wish to know.

The debate on genetic testing for insurance purposes is only just beginning but the common concerns about coercion and confidentiality are already being expressed. There is also concern that enthusiasm for genetic screening considerably exceeds current knowledge of its utility and rational interpretation of its results. Guide-lines which are legally binding on the insurance industry will be necessary to protect applicants' interests and to ensure scrupulous practice on the part of the insurance companies.

DNA fingerprinting

DNA fingerprinting, like traditional fingerprinting, offers a means of identifying individual people because every DNA fingerprint is unique to a person, with the exception of twins. A fingerprint can be obtained from very small samples of blood, hair, skin, or other biological materials using PCR amplification techniques. The use of DNA fingerprinting in criminal investigations, or civil proceedings, such as paternity suits, can therefore be very valuable. However, before subjecting a person to an invasive technique such as the taking of blood or even the extraction of hair that person's written consent should be sought. This is not only good ethical practice but is also important for legal reasons: if someone were to carry out either procedure against a person's wishes he or she might risk an action for battery.

The need for consent to samples being taken for DNA fingerprinting was reaffirmed in a recent paternity suit, in Scotland. A putative father of an illegitimate child refused to give blood for DNA testing. The mother's lawyer applied for a court order to compel him to do so but the application was denied both by the Sheriff court and on appeal. A further appeal to the Scottish Court of Session also failed, the judge ruling that to compel a defendant to an invasive procedure which he does not want and which would help build the case of the plaintiff 'offends the principle of fairness on which Scottish law is based'. A question this case raises is whether the courts would have been more likely to waive the need for consent for a less invasive procedure such as the taking of a hair sample. Furthermore, could an individual reasonably refuse to give such a sample? Such decisions might depend on the extent to which it would be in the child's interests to have the issue of paternity settled. These issues are more likely to be resolved as specific cases set legal precedents.

Despite the obvious benefits of DNA fingerprinting, its use still raises moral concerns. Many people fear that blood samples taken for one use may also be used to obtain a fingerprint without a person's knowledge. A national database has even been proposed which would hold a DNA fingerprint of all new-born babies. The police, in addition, have suggested recently that a DNA sample be obtained from every man (but not woman) in the country, an idea apparently supported by a government select committee. The reason for holding such information would ostensibly be to help in the capture of rapists, murderers, and other criminals but the potential for the information to be used for more underhand reasons is substantial. The idea of a government routinely gaining such powerful, identifying information without any specific reason is likely to give rise to public concern. The use of DNA fingerprinting therefore will need to be carefully regulated to ensure that society only benefits from its application and that the privacy of the public is protected.

Eugenics

The term 'eugenics' is one which historically has provoked, and continues to provoke, strong emotional reactions. The common response has a great deal to do with the lengths to which the Nazis went in their attempts to produce a 'racially purified' Aryan population. While it is understandable that potential parents may make careful choices in their selection of a mate, it is entirely different for other people deliberately to try to ensure that some couples do, and others do not, reproduce; particularly if those efforts involve any pressure or compulsion upon potential parents.

The term 'eugenics' was coined and introduced in the late nineteenth century by the English mathematician Francis Galton. He derived it from the Greek word meaning 'well-born'. Galton defined eugenics as the science of improving the human population through 'judicious matings ... to give the more suitable races or strains of blood a better chance of prevailing speedily over the less suitable'. As Suzuki and Knudtson observe in their book *Genethics*, that characterization of eugenics exhibits 'a candour seldom encountered amongst adherents of modern eugenics'.

Galton's ideas, and those of other eugenicists, received influential and powerful support in some sections of American society, with the result that in the early part of this century some thirty American states passed laws requiring the compulsory sterilization of certain groups of individuals, typically those categorized as, for example, the 'feebleminded', epileptic, and mentally ill. The legislation was never comprehensively enforced, but many thousands of people were compulsorily sterilized, mostly in the state of California.

Nazi Germany exhibited the most offensive and ruthless commitment to eugenicist ideas. The rationalization which the Nazis invoked for their appalling treatment of Jews, gypsies, homosexuals, and people with mental illnesses or handicaps relied heavily on eugenicist theories. The use of ideas purporting to have a scientific, and particularly a genetic, basis for unforgivable acts of oppression and brutality has understandably created a situation in which all and any proposals to influence, manipulate, or control the genetic characteristics of human populations will, and should, be scrutinized with immense care, and no small measure of scepticism.

Using the science of genetic modification to produce a 'master race', or to select children with particular attributes, is unacceptable. Even if parents are entirely free to reproduce as they choose, considerable social and ethical problems could arise if we eventually reach the currently remote possibility of being able to choose not just the gender but also some of the physical, emotional, and intellectual attributes of our children. If it became commonplace, for example, for parents to choose a boy as their first child, then this might well make it even harder to diminish sexual discrimination in our society.

Chapter Fourteen

The Implications of the Human Genome Project

The Project

The ambitious aim of the Human Genome Project (HGP) is to map the positions of all the genes in the human genome. Molecular genetics had by the 1970s reached the stage at which scientists could sequence perhaps 100 base pairs per year. By the mid-1980s a single scientist could identify 10,000 to 20,000 bases a year. By 1985 a cumulative total of about 2,000,000 bases had been sequenced.

Substantial though that achievement may have been, it falls a long way short of the three billion base pairs which will have to be identified for the HGP to be completed. Experimental techniques continue to improve but the magnitude of the task of sequencing should not be underestimated. One problem with estimating how long the task will take is that there is no agreement about the size of the human genome. One estimate is that there are about 100,000 genes, of which so far 4 per cent have been located, but even these have not been sequenced. According to one estimate, to complete the full project would cost about 30,000 person years of scientifically skilled labour. That is, of course, equivalent to 3,000 scientists and technicians working for an entire decade.

A debate on the HGP

By comparison with most other countries in which a contribution is actively being made to the HGP, there has been very little debate in the UK on its merits and likely consequences. Unfortunately, the few critical comments which have been made have often been misinterpreted as if they were attacks on science in general. Such a confusion is undesirable, though it is perhaps explicable. Many research scientists in British universities consider that public sector funding policies have left their research in a vulnerable and beleaguered condition. Consequently they may fear that any suggestion that money might be better spent is liable to be interpreted as an argument that money should be taken away from scientific research rather than redistributed to other scientific projects.

The same considerations might explain why it is that in the USA, criticism of the cost and pace of the HGP are usually taken as specific criticisms of that particular project. It would be desirable therefore if the limited and relatively private debate on the relative virtues of the HGP when compared to other scientific priorities could be conducted in Britain in the public arena.

The case for and against the HGP

One of the leading American enthusiasts for the HGP, the molecular biologist Walter Gilbert has said that 'The total human sequence is the grail of human genetics' (Suzuki and Knudtson 1990). For its advocates and supporters the completion of the HGP is expected to enable answers to be given to all the important questions in human genetics, and to establish a basis from which all human genetic problems can be solved.

Completing the HGP would certainly shift the focus of research from trying to locate the genes to finding out what they actually do. According to some commentators, this is going to do far more for science than it will for medical practice. It would be premature to contemplate settling a debate of that kind, but it does indicate that medical practitioners cannot take for granted that the completion of the

HGP will have a substantial impact on clinical practice. Nevertheless, it cannot be disputed that there will be some benefits for medicine: as the genome is sequenced, more disease-related genes are likely to be revealed which will in turn allow new carrier, presymptomatic, or pre-natal tests to be developed. Also, as the sequences of hormones and other proteins are clarified it will become possible to produce new pharmaceutical products for the treatment of hereditary illnesses, using similar techniques to those already employed for cloning human insulin and human growth hormone.

The direct relevance of completing the HGP to scientific biology is relatively easy to perceive. It might, for example, make it far easier to clarify the evolutionary relationships between humans and other species, but only once the genomes of those other species had also been sequenced. It might, furthermore, provide what might be termed 'a molecular clock' with which to measure the passage of evolutionary time. When the project has been completed we should have far more information with which to answer the question to what extent people are genetically equal. The relative significance of genetics and the environment to the development of characteristics continues to be debated, but a case could be made for adjourning some of those arguments until the HGP enables us to know with some accuracy just how relevant genetics may be with respect to the contested topics. A related debate has been concerned not with the differences between people, but with establishing the extent to which genes do, or do not, in general limit the abilities and options of human beings. The completion of the HGP might introduce some clarity to that debate too. It is, however, even at this stage very difficult to know precisely how informative the completion of the HGP will be.

Those commentators who are most sceptical about the practical, and especially the medical, utility of the HGP argue that by no means all human health problems are fundamentally genetic in character. They maintain, on the contrary, that genetics seems to be directly relevant to only a minority of the most urgent conditions. Consequently they suggest that there is a potential risk that investing substantial resources into the HGP may unduly inhibit other desirable and valuable scientific and medical research projects.

The cost of the HGP

Estimates of the eventual cost of completing the HGP vary. Producing reliable estimates is very difficult. If resources are poured into the HGP we can expect to achieve some economies of scale. On the other hand, as time passes experimental techniques can be expected to improve, and therefore by working at a slower pace we might considerably lower the total cost. One estimate suggests that if the HGP were to be completed within ten years, the total cost might be in the order of three billion US dollars.

When faced with a call on funding of that magnitude, critics will emphasize what economists term 'the opportunity costs' of investing such a large quantity of money into one project. Opportunity costs are supposed to represent the value of other activities which cannot be undertaken as a result of making a specific investment decision. If three billion dollars go into the HGP, that may be counted as three billions less for other potentially attractive projects.

The enthusiasts for the HGP respond to that argument by predicting very substantial returns to that admittedly relatively high level of investment. They can also plausibly argue that most of the money coming to the HGP is not an opportunity cost to other scientific projects but rather represents extra spending on science which might otherwise not be made. It is quite likely that the remarkable achievement involved in galvanizing sufficient support and funding to launch the HGP means that at least some of its funding should be counted as additional monies which would not otherwise be available to science. The Department of Education and Science has agreed to provide the Medical Research Council (MRC) with an extra £11m over three years (1989–1992) to support the UK's contribution to the HGP. That money is on top of its science quota to the MRC of approximately £110m per year. The decision to provide that commitment was taken at the very highest level of the British government.

Economic grounds have not, however, been the only basis from which commentators have criticized the HGP; philosophical considerations have also been invoked. One line of argument has been that the pursuit of the HGP is predicated upon a set of implausible and unreliable assumptions about the relevance of genetics to human biology. Genetics is seen by some commentators as incorrigibly reductionist, and those critics tend to argue, in effect, that the biological whole is sometimes more than merely the sum of its parts. Anti-reductionists emphasize, for example, that atoms exhibit properties which cannot be represented or explained as merely the sum of the properties of the individual elementary particles of which atoms are composed. Similarly, molecules exhibit so-called emergent properties not found amongst atoms, cells have properties not found amongst molecules, and organisms have properties which exceed those properties characteristic of cells.

These are issues which are philosophical rather than empirical, but they comprise various standpoints from which differing protagonists approach the HGP. While it is not possible in this context to resolve any of those philosophical debates, scientists who are sceptical about the extent to which human biology can be reduced to human genetics can, and do, point to observations such as the fact that even identical twins who have indistinguishable genetic fingerprints, nonetheless have different skin fingerprints. That fact is not remotely conclusive, but does indicate that at least some facts of human biology which might at first sight seem to be genetically determined cannot be accounted for in purely genetic terms.

Given that the HGP is already under way, rather than querying the wisdom of its creation, it may well be more appropriate to consider the practical question about the best way in which it should be pursued and applied. In so far as public funds are being devoted to the HGP, it would seem reasonable to expect that those resources should be targeted in the first place either on those conditions which afflict a relatively large number of people rather than the rarer conditions, or on sequencing the genes responsible for the most serious clinical distress.

Problems for the HGP

One of the scientifically most intriguing, and medically most significant, questions facing molecular genetics is whether all, most, or some of the entire human genome is biologically important. The dominant school of thought subscribes to the view that a large number of the base-pair sequences in the human genome carry no significant genetic information at all. From this position such putatively insignificant sequences are typically referred to as 'junk DNA'. If much of the human genome is junk, or genetically vacuous, then nothing will be gained by sequencing it. According to that view, the most sensible research strategy would be to distinguish all the junk DNA from the authentic genes, and then concentrate on the latter while ignoring the former. Given that the repeated execution of procedures to sequence DNA is scientifically unchallenging and may even be rather dull, many geneticists would be delighted if only a modest fraction of the entire genome actually deserved to be sequenced.

Not all scientists, however, accept the hypothesis implicit in the concept of junk DNA. For example, Gilbert has suggested that any characterization of some DNA sequences as junk might merely be a reflection of our current ignorance about their true function. He proposes, therefore, that the entire human genome should be sequenced, in part to help the scientific community learn precisely what the functions are of those portions currently disparaged as junk. The hypothesis that they may have uses which we have not identified can certainly not yet be refuted. If, as some scientists suspect, only a small proportion of all genes are involved in the aetiology of human diseases, would it not be extravagant or even wasteful to devote resources to sequencing maybe 100,000 genes, not to mention the putative junk? No one is yet in a position to know which approach will turn out to have been correct, but the debate is obviously of more than purely academic interest. The extent of public support for science would hardly be enhanced if a large portion of a large sum were devoted to sequencing a great deal of DNA of no scientific or medical significance. On the other hand, it might be wasteful only to sequence those parts of the human genome which are already known to be important, if segments not currently thought to be important were subsequently shown to be vital.

It would appear that a consensus is emerging in both the USA and the UK to begin by mapping the genome as a basis for deciding which sections to sequence, rather than sequencing the entire genome starting at the very beginning and continuing to the very end. While there may be such a consensus, there is no unanimity. The policy in the UK is to map those parts of the genome which are already known or believed to be functional, that is to say those parts which are known to be expressed as proteins. Given the present state of our knowledge and the scale of available funding, that would seem to be a sensible choice.

The contribution of private funding for the HGP

Both public and private sources of funding have long made separate and complementary contributions to the support of scientific and technological research and development, but the funding of the HGP, especially in the USA, has occasioned a more vigorous debate about the roles of the public and private sectors, especially in relation to the potential exploitation of the product of that research.

Walter Gilbert argues that the HGP can and should be substantially funded and exploited by the private sector. While no one is arguing that the private sector has, or should have, no part to play in the HGP, many commentators have expressed serious concern about the possible consequences which might arise if the dissemination and exploitation of the results of the HGP were unduly subordinated to commercial considerations.

In the USA the Genome Corporation, and several other similarly motivated companies such as Collaborative Research, view their research in essentially commercial terms. That is not to suggest that they do not expect it to contribute to general social welfare, but their approach is commercial rather than charitable.

In order to persuade private sector investors to place their profit-seeking funds with human genome research companies rather than with competitive alternatives, the private commercial genome researchers have to be in a position to forecast substantial profits. Those prospective profits can only be generated under a specific set of restricted conditions. Not merely would those firms need to map and sequence human genes, but they would need to sequence them ahead of any competitors, and then be in a position to market their results at commercially advantageous prices. It is this fact which is provoking considerable concern and a vigorous debate, because some commentators fear that the prices which would be charged, or which may need to be charged if normal commercial rates of return are to be achieved, may be so high that the full potential clinical benefits of mapping and sequencing the genome will either not be achieved, will be achieved far too slowly, or will become available only to those able to meet the relatively high costs involved.

Gilbert has defended his commercial approach to the HGP by arguing, in part, that sequencing the human genome would not actually be a research project at all, but rather a biotechnology production-line job. According to this line of argument, it is more like routine cartography than pioneering exploration. That claim has some plausibility, but is more a prediction than it is a description. It presupposes that pursuing the HGP will provoke a range of technological improvements in the techniques of molecular biology, so that the degree of experimental skill required to complete the work will decline, making it a routinized process rather than cutting edge research.

The key issue in this debate is whether or not a scientifically and ethically responsible approach to the application of the results of the HGP is compatible with the demands of commercial profitability. Many take the view that it is not. For example, Robert Cook-Deegan, an analyst at the Office of Technology Assessment, has been quoted as having said: 'If a company behaves in what scientists believe is a socially responsible manner, they can't make a profit' (Roberts 1987). This is probably an extreme view; it is to be hoped that the choice between responsibility and profit is not so stark. The important thing is getting a balance which achieves the maximum benefit of the project with the minimum concomitant harm. It is possible that some degree of commercial profitability may help stimulate the work, thus increasing benefits. Profitability does, however, rely on the ownership of information. This would require copyrighting or patenting of the human genome. In the next section we consider the considerable problems posed by patenting and copyrighting.

Copyrighting and patenting the human genome

If private sector research-based corporations are to transform the results of their human genome research into a marketable product two main potential strategies suggest themselves: they might try either to copyright or to patent the sequences which they decode. Patenting is, in general, a far stronger claim to ownership than copyrighting. When something has been copyrighted, a payment is only due on its reproduction, not for its application. If you publish a book of non-fiction, people infringe your copyright if they try to sell reproductions of your text, but if they use the information which you have published they do not have to pay you a licence fee. If, for example, a team of scientists were to identify and sequence the gene for blue eyes, they would hold the copyright on its subsequent publication, and might also seek to patent it. If they only held the copyright, they would not be able to claim a licence fee if someone used the results of their work to enable parents to have blue-eyed children. If they were granted a patent, however, such a licence fee would then become payable.

Patenting the human genome

The question of whether or not a patent could be claimed on sections of the human genome has never yet been answered formally. An occasion on which a decision would have to be made has not yet arisen, and the authorities have issued no definitive guidance on the matter. For many people, the idea of patenting the human genome is morally objectionable. They question how a company could have rights over something which is inherent in every individual and argue that the human genome should be owned by nobody. If it were to be possible however, the commercial incentives for private investment would be relatively more attractive. Even so it is by no means obvious that sufficient returns could be generated to compensate for the massive quantities of capital which would be required, nor for the time which might intervene between when the investment might be made and when the returns start to arrive.

Some have argued that, despite the historical tradition of not allowing the patenting of human beings, or parts of human beings, the scope of patents should be expanded to include some or all of the human genome. Those who argue in favour of patenting human genetic sequences do not maintain merely that a commercial incentive is required if scientists are to pursue their researches, for that argument is an entirely general one and applies to most, if not all, science-based high technology research and cannot by itself justify extending patent rights into an area from which tradition has always assumed that it would be excluded. They also argue, specifically, that the gene sequence is not something which can readily be known, but on the contrary that in order to make it accessible and comprehensible researchers need to develop and apply biochemical machines and computer programmes which will be both expensive and in themselves patentable. They argue that the discoveries derived from such equipment, analyses, and efforts should also belong to the individuals and organization concerned. They are arguing, in effect, that despite the fact that the sequence will not be unique to any particular individual, it will be the unique product of the skills involved in mapping and sequencing it. Even if that latter argument were to be valid, it is not by itself an argument for patenting rather than, for example, copyright protection.

In the UK, patent law is sufficiently ambiguous that it is difficult to know whether or not the Patent Office would accept an application for a human genome patent. Even if a patent were not granted in the UK, some other country might see fit to take such a novel step, and then the problem of international recognition would arise. Whatever the rights or wrongs of those arguments may be, it is generally recognized that the rules of patent priority and those which govern the recognition of scientific priority may, and almost certainly will, conflict. In the UK, the rules governing the award of patents specify that prior disclosure of the substance of an application will undermine the validity of any application. Such a rule goes against established and accepted principles of scientific practice. It is not that all members of the scientific community always obey those principles, but in so far as they conceal their methods, evidence, or conclusions they undermine the proper functioning of the scientific world. While a minority of scientists might see it as in their short-term interests to act secretively, it is against the long-term interests of science as a whole that such non-cooperative practices should spread. The problem of disclosure undermining a patent application has been overcome in the USA and Japan by establishing a period of grace during which disclosure might occur without prejudice to a subsequent application for a patent. The UK has still to resolve the issue.

If it is genuinely the case that the HGP has a great deal to offer to clinical practice, then the failure to reveal the results of the sequences at the earliest possible moment would be directly disadvantageous to potential patients, and therefore to public health. If, furthermore, sequences are to be covered by patent protection, then the costs of any subsequent clinical applications will inevitably be higher than might otherwise be the case and, under conditions of restricted funding, they will almost certainly mean that such benefits as may accrue will be available more slowly and to fewer patients than the optimum number.

The rules which govern the granting of patents could undermine science in yet another way. It is hard to gain a patent unless the application names only a small and tightly restricted list of individuals, whereas a scientific paper from a multidisciplinary team, of the sort which typically works on the HGP, will be characterized by lengthy lists of multiple authors.

For both moral and practical reasons, therefore, it would not be appropriate to allow the patenting of some or all of the human genome. However, the idea of copyrighting sequences of the human genome might be regarded more favourably.

Copyrighting the human genome

Many of the same kinds of commercial considerations which have been invoked to defend the suggestion of patenting the human genome could be, and have been, articulated in defence of the possibility of copyright claims. The directors of the Genome Corporation have told potential investors that they intend to apply for, and obtain, the copyright on each and every sequence they identify. While the legal questions concerning the patenting of the human genome remain unresolved, lawyers working for the US Office of Technology Assessment, which advises Congress, concluded in 1987 that US law would permit parts, or all, of the human genome to be copyrighted. The corresponding positions under UK law and that of the European Community have yet to be clarified.

Precisely how the device of copyrighting might apply in this context is also unclear. The key question concerns the extent to which the copyrighted material is, or is not, in the public domain, and the consequent restrictions which may be placed upon its use. The protection afforded by copyrighting normally applies in a straightforward fashion to the publication of scientific books and papers. It is not obvious that those who want to copyright sequences of the human genome have that standard model in mind, or something rather different and more like a patent.

If books and papers specifying the base sequence of human genes are published then the authors should undoubtedly expect at least the same copyright protection as is given for example, to the publishers of this volume. In that event, individuals and organizations, other than the authors, will not be prevented from using all and any of the information that the copyrighted database provides; they will only be prevented from making an exact copy for commercial resale.

Gilbert's reported position is not entirely clear. He has been quoted as having said that 'researchers will have to pay a fee to use it just as they have to pay a fee when they use the information they obtain in a scientific journal. That fee is the cover price.' (McKie 1988: p. 115.) But it is not obvious that the analogy with a cover price can be appropriate. When scientists buy their journals, the cover price is intended to enable the publishers to recoup the costs of running the journal (i.e. the costs of the editorial office and staff, plus paper, printing, and distribution costs), but it is not intended to compensate either the publisher or the authors for the costs incurred in conducting the research which underlies the scientific papers.

From a strictly commercial point of view, copyrighting is the inappropriate model to describe what private non-charitable investors would want or expect. Authors can only copyright what they publish, and if a human gene sequence is published it will be available in any and every scientific library. But if the scientists who discover the sequence, or their employers, insist on selling copies of the sequence only directly to final users in exchange for a fee, that would not amount to publishing it, in the way that scientific publications are normally made publicly available. It would be more like the sale of a secret commercial report.

If the results of all human genome research are published in a normal journal format which all universities, colleges, or public libraries can buy at a price which reflects the costs of production of the publication, then the authors will have, and will properly be entitled to, copyright. But if they ask for a fee for applying the sequence as opposed to just reading it, then they are not trying to obtain the copyright, but something closer to patent protection. The argument is not about whether or not there should be a price for the publication containing the results of the genome project, but it is about the level at which prices may be set, and the market in which those prices are determined. If the price is set so as to recoup the costs of research then it cannot amount to publishing, but would merely be the confidential sale of privileged information.

A company engaged in the HGP as a commercial venture would have every incentive to charge a price for their information which would be as high as the market could possibly stand. But if they endeavoured to maximize the returns on their investment then what they would be doing should not be counted as publishing, and their commercial protection would lie not in the legislation of copyrighting but normal commercial confidentiality. Under those circumstances, however, the price is likely to be so prohibitively high as effectively to prevent non-commercial medical authorities from being able to obtain and apply the information to their clinical practice. The only arrangements which might make economic sense for commercial genome mapping companies would not make medical sense. Medical science and clinical care would benefit most from the straightforward publication of all the results of the HGP as soon as they became available, under conditions which would preclude charges being made for their application; but under those conditions it is difficult to envisage commercial genome research being economically viable.

In order to try to maximize the returns on their investment, commercial genome companies would probably try to persuade industrial employers and insurance companies to require genetic screening tests for their employees and customers. Any initiatives taken along those lines might be expected to provoke the sorts of problems which were outlined in the previous chapter in connection with genetic screening.

The evident enthusiasm for privatizing the results of the HGP have not remained uncontested. An unidentified American scientist has been quoted as having, rather bluntly, said: 'This knowledge belongs to mankind—not to a bunch of boardroom financiers. In any case, all the groundwork has been funded by public research bodies and medical charities. It is not right that private firms should now try to reap the benefits.' (McKie 1988: p. 110.) More generally, many commentators have argued that since the human genome is a collective biological property of the entire human race, it should correspondingly be designated as collective economic property.

What some have seen as a reasonable compromise between the interests of particular teams of scientific researchers and the collective interests of science as a whole has been instituted in France by the Centre d'Étude du Polymorphisme Humain (CEPH). The centre allows researchers to use its materials with the proviso that they, in turn, send their data back to CEPH. Researchers will still benefit from some proprietory protection as they may request that their materials should not be made public for one year, although they will be available to other CEPH collaborators. With an arrangement of that type, scientists are able to co-operate more freely while still keeping intact the mechanisms for awarding recognition for scientific originality and leaving the opportunity for a group of discoverers to market an industrial application of their discovery ahead of potential competitors. In the UK, researchers whose projects are funded by the Medical Research

Council must deposit their results in a database which is available to all.

Privatizing the results of the HGP

There is no law to prohibit the investment of private resources into the HGP, and any proposal for such legislation would be unreasonable, but from the investors' point of view it will probably be an extremely risky venture. From the point of view of those people whose health might benefit from the applications of that research, contributions to the funding of research should be welcomed as long as they are intended charitably rather than commercially. In so far as the HGP is a commercial project there is an unavoidable risk that the consequent restrictions, operating for example through a price mechanism, upon the dissemination and availability of the results will almost certainly prevent some people benefiting from the application of the knowledge which would otherwise be publicly available.

A further problem which might arise from the privatization of HGP research is that there may be a gratuitous and wasteful duplication of effort, which could otherwise be avoided. Duplication is not always wasteful. There is some evidence that if just two or three groups are working in the same field it can encourage scientists to work harder and faster than they otherwise might. But if the number of competing teams rises beyond a low figure, then wasteful duplication is unavoidable. Healthy competition can and should be achieved without resorting to the commercialization of research into public health.

The interest of patients, and of the National Health Service, will best be served if HGP research is pursued either in public laboratories with public funds, or with private funding of a charitable nature. The results of all such work should, moreover, be publicly available to the entire scientific community in precisely the same way as the results of other medical research projects, and charges should not be levied for the application of the results of the HGP. The priorities within the HGP should be set so as to maximize therapeutic benefits as part of a global effort to reduce the suffering from genetically transmitted illnesses.

Chapter Fifteen

Summary and Conclusions

General

The techniques of genetic modification have the potential, through application in agriculture, medicine, and technology, to increase the well-being of people and to promote the health of the population by disease prevention. Wrongly used, they also have the potential to cause harm. We believe that, as is the case with other forms of technology, genetic modification in itself is neither good nor bad, but care must be taken to optimize the benefits and minimize the risks it offers. In our opinion, those developing the techniques and applications of the new technology have a duty to consider the consequences of their activities, and careful consideration must be given by the scientific community to this issue. We recommend that scientific bodies such as the Royal Society, organizations funding research in this field such as the Research Councils, and coordinating centres such as the Human Genome Project devote greater resources and efforts to consideration of the ethical, social, and environmental implications of developments in this field.

Public education

People's lack of knowledge about genetic modification has in the past given rise to fear and to opposition to new developments. We believe that these fears are largely unfounded, but that combating them by adopting a paternalistic or secretive approach is not the answer. Instead, the scientific community, both in academia and commerce, has a duty to inform the general public of new developments in the applications of genetic modification in a manner comprehensible to lay people. Schools, radio, television and publishers of books, journals, and newspapers also have an important role to play in achieving this end.

The BMA would actively support medical and scientific experts working with schools, colleges, universities, and the various media to bring to the attention of the public the scientific, social, and ethical implications of genetic modification. Furthermore, we recognize the extensive work of the European Community in examining these issues but would urge the Commission to consider adopting an action plan which would bring the discussion more into the public arena.

Medical education

Medical education does not at present give sufficient weight to the ethical aspects of the practice of medicine and we recommend that the link between the ethics and practice of medicine be incorporated at every stage of medical education.

There is evidence that understanding among members of the medical profession of genetics and of genetic disease is insufficient. Medical schools, the Royal Colleges and the General Medical Council (GMC) are urged to take action to improve the understanding among all health disciplines of the science and ethics of genetic modification, the principles and methods of genetic counselling, and the implications of genetic disease. We consider that these areas should be included in examinations, and that post-qualification education should be encouraged.

Food

It is probable that food products or ingredients derived from genetic modification of micro-organisms, plants, and animals will become increasingly common. Stringent safety precautions must be adopted during the development of such products and the subsequent marketing and distribution of the products need to be carefully monitored.

Consumers ought to be informed when food products contain genetically modified ingredients. Such foods therefore should be appropriately labelled. If the use of genetic modification in food products is treated in an open manner, consumer confidence is likely to increase, leading to a more rapid acceptance of the new techniques.

Bacteria and viruses

In our opinion, no ethical problems are associated with the genetic modification of bacteria and viruses per se. However, indiscriminate release of bacteria or viruses might have the potential to cause major environmental change. It is vital therefore that before any release, a proper and rigorous assessment of the likely consequences be made. If it is decided to release the microbes, the actual effect of the release must be monitored, and the predicted consequences compared with the reality in order to improve predictions of the consequences of subsequent releases.

The release of genetically modified bacteria and viruses in the form of live vaccines should be carefully controlled. At present the construction of the vaccines is covered by the Health and Safety Executive (HSE) while the marketing of the vaccines is controlled by the Medicines Control Agency of the Department of Health. Under new regulations to come in to effect in 1992 the construction of, testing (trials), and marketing of live vaccines will come under the authority of both the HSE and Department of Environment with the Department of Health playing only an advisory role. We do not support the weakening of the role of the DoH in the regulation of genetically modified vaccines and recommend that the three agencies have equal powers in decisions about the use of live vaccines.

Plants

The recommendation concerning the release of bacteria and viruses (see above) would apply similarly to plants.

We are concerned that companies involved in the production of herbicides could potentially become involved in the development of herbicide-resistant crops. We recognize that these companies have a commercial interest in promoting increased use of herbicides and that this may be made easier if resistant crops are developed. There should be no increase in the amount of herbicides used, if it is not justified by need, and we recommend that the regulatory authorities should not permit the introduction of herbicide-resistant strains if this leads to undesirable increases in the use of herbicides.

Animals

Production of animals by genetic modification does not give rise to new ethical considerations, but, as in any research using animals, the degree of suffering induced as a result of genetic modification has to be weighed against potential for benefit.

The production of new transgenic animal models to study human diseases (e.g. oncomouse) is controlled by the Home Office under the Animal (Scientific Procedures) Act 1986. However, we question whether doctors and veterinary surgeons, as Home Office Inspectors, should be the sole arbiters in deciding what is ethical and in approving Project Licences. There should be more room for public debate in these matters and we would urge that the role of the Animals Procedures Committee, an advisory body with small representation from animal welfare organizations, be expanded to include the routine assessment of all animal research protocols before they receive approval from the Inspectorate. Currently, the Committee sees very few Project Licences and is not routinely asked to comment on research protocols involving genetically modified animals. We would also urge greater representation of animal welfare groups on the Committee.

It is important that bio-diversity of both commercial and wild species is maintained. This ideally should be achieved by maintaining large groups of animals in their natural habitats. We are not persuaded that maintenance of bio-diversity can properly be accomplished through private enterprise. The establishment of national gene banks is one way in which genetic diversity can be maintained, but it is not enough.

We deplore the practice of unauthorized removal of plants and animals from developing countries with subsequent exploitation of the genetic material and without return of benefit to the source country.

People

Human genetic modification should be restricted to treatment or prevention of serious disease. Somatic cell gene therapy should be used only when there is no other alternative available or when it offers genuine advantages, such as safety or efficacy, over other types of treatment. With these reservations, we believe that somatic cell gene therapy has considerable potential. We do not consider that it poses any novel ethical problems.

Germ-line gene therapy would cause changes not only to the genetic make-up of an individual but also to his or her descendants. It is possible that the consequences of such changes, whether due to damage during the modification process or to the loss of a gene with hidden advantages from the gene pool, may not become apparent for several generations. We consider that germ-line gene therapy would benefit only a very small number of people, as in many conditions alternatives to germ-line gene therapy, such as preimplantation diagnosis, are already available. It is probable that over the next few years the techniques of embryo screening will advance to cover an increased number of conditions. We feel strongly that since the risks associated with germ-line gene therapy are potentially so great, our expertise is so limited, and the number of people for whom it seems to offer the only treatment is so small, this type of therapy is not justifiable either now or for the foreseeable future.

Genetic screening, whether carrier, diagnostic, or pre-natal, should always be accompanied by non-directive counselling. It should be on a strictly voluntary basis (an exception would be screening children for PKU) and confidential. If a person should refuse to accept screening for whatever reason it should not jeopardize either that person's rights, or his or her children's rights, to subsequent care or state benefits.

National screening programmes should be established only for diseases where treatment, or termination in the case of pre-natal screening, is available or where a positive test result will give people information on which to base life-changing decisions (for example whether or not to have children).

We consider that sex selection for sex-linked diseases is acceptable. However, we would urge continuing research into the development of disease-specific diagnostic tests in order to prevent unnecessary termination of healthy fetuses. We believe it is inappropriate for doctors to offer sex selection 'treatments' to couples for non-medical reasons.

Use of genetic information

Genetic screening for certain diseases or predispositions may be appropriate in some workplace settings, subject to certain restrictions. The tests must be accurate and the link between a positive test result and the risk of developing a subsequent health problem must be unequivocally established before any routine testing is carried out. However, it must be borne in mind that some types of work involve a significant risk of morbidity through accident or industrial disease. The potential contribution of susceptibility to genetic disease to the overall risk should be taken into account when workplace screening is considered.

The rationale behind workplace screening must always be to

provide the individual with information relevant to the promotion and maintenance of his or her health. It should not be used to exclude people from employment, or to avoid the implementation of safer working practices or working environment. Employees or prospective employees must have the right to refuse genetic screening without prejudice to their employment prospects.

We do not believe that insurance companies are justified in carrying out genetic screening at present. The major killer diseases such as cardiovascular disease and cancer are affected not only by genetic susceptibility, but also by many other factors such as diet and exercise. In addition, the link between genetic markers and development of these diseases is not sufficiently well established to permit the accurate prediction of actuarial risk. Although it is possible that some individuals may choose to take out or increase existing insurance cover on learning by means of genetic screening that they have an increased susceptibility to developing serious disease, we feel that it is better for everyone to pay higher premiums than to put some people into the position of having to undergo tests against their wishes.

The taking of samples for DNA fingerprinting should be carried out only with the consent of the individual. Doctors must not participate in the obtaining of samples without consent. During a criminal investigation, only the DNA profiles of those found guilty may be retained in police records. All profiles obtained from innocent people must be destroyed. Profiles obtained for medical or civil reasons must not be transferred to any other data-bank. The establishment, for forensic reasons, of central databases containing DNA profiles of entire populations or groups would not be acceptable.

We consider that information about an individual's genetic make-up obtained for medical reasons, like other medical data, should be treated as confidential. However, we recognize that difficulties may arise concerning confidentiality within families when other family members may have an interest in knowing a relation's genetic make-up.

Regulation

We recommend that the regulation of genetic modification be conducted in an open, democratically accountable and representative fashion. The views of different interest groups including legislators, ethicists, scientists, health and environmental experts, and the general public should be taken into account.

Established recommendations must be effectively enforced. We recommend that a properly funded inspectorate should be established to monitor adherence to registration requirements.

It is important to take into account socio-economic, ethical, and environmental implications when considering approval of products involving the use of genetic modification and we therefore believe that the introduction of a 'fourth hurdle' is appropriate. We would support the extension of the 'fourth hurdle' to products manufactured by conventional means.

The early caution shown by scientists working in the field of genetic modification is commendable. Despite the criticism levelled by some commentators, we feel that their careful approach has done no harm in the long run, and has enabled the potential risks of genetic modification to be considered at length. We would like to see more self-regulation of this type among scientists.

The cautious approach to release of genetically modified organisms is likewise correct. The use of the 'sophisticated trial and error' approach, erring on the side of caution, should be continued. In our opinion, it is vital that the consequences of the release of such organisms should be considered carefully and dispassionately by a release committee.

Health and safety

The HSE, while carrying responsibility for the safety of laboratory workers, lacks financial and personnel resources. In addition, the penalties levied against companies whose lax health and safety standards result in injuries and deaths are insufficient. We strongly recommend that the resources of the HSE be strengthened and that the penalties for infringing safety law be increased.

Safety training in university laboratories is frequently unsatisfactory and carried out on an *ad hoc* basis. National guide-lines on training for work with bio-hazards, genetically modified organisms, and other potential threats to the individual or to the environment should be established by funding bodies or scientific societies. A formal system of training researchers and students should be introduced.

Patenting and copyrighting

The issue of patenting is complex and important. We believe that it would be premature to adopt the European Commission's draft Directive on patenting without a fuller and more public exploration of the issues involved. At present, conflicting interpretations of the Directive have been made, including one that the Directive would in effect permit patenting of not only genetically modified but also naturally occurring plants and animals which had not previously been described. We do not believe that living organisms should be patented and urge the European Commission to oppose any relaxation of regulations which would result in such patents being permitted. The practices in the USA should not be allowed to influence unduly the nature of legislation in Europe, and we would prefer the European Patent Convention to be retained.

We take the view that patenting of the DNA sequences constituting the human genome is ethically unacceptable. We urge all those involved in this field of research, particularly those responsible for the HGP, to resist commercial pressures towards patenting. The results of human genome work should be freely available and should not be treated as a marketable commodity.

Fears have been expressed that, as a consequence of the establishment of such requirements, private venture capital may be discouraged from investing in human genome research.

If that is the case, and if it is still considered that the project should be funded, public money must be made available. We feel strongly that the issues raised are too fundamental for decisions to be dictated by the pressures of commercial companies.

We consider that the profits available to private companies from utilizing information on the human genome will be sufficient to permit them to fund genome research without the added financial incentive of obtaining patents.

Copyrighting is acceptable, provided that it fits into the established practice of publishing papers in the scientific press. We believe that any attempt to cover the costs of research by charging a high price for published work and restricting its distribution would be inappropriate. However, while we believe that the identity of the human genome is the collective property of the whole human race, we consider that an acceptable compromise between dissemination of knowledge and the protection of researchers has been found by the CEPH. Those responsible for the organization of the HGP should consider supporting the establishment of a similar system.

Funding research

Central government should increase the funds available for pure research in the field of human genetics. This will have the effect of broadening the research base and will reduce the influence of private companies with a financial stake in promoting developments in a particular area.

Given the potential expense of the HGP, we support the present trend of mapping the sections which seem to offer most benefit, to be followed in time with studies on other parts of the genome.

REFERENCES

BAINBRIDGE, B. W. (1987), *Genetics of Microbes* (2nd edn.), Blackie.

BAIRD, P. A., ANDERSON, T. W., NEWCOMBE, H. B., and LOWRY, R. B. (1988), 'Genetic disorders in children and young adults: a population study', *American Journal of Human Genetics*, 42: 677–93.

BLOOM, B. R. (1989), 'Vaccines for the Third World', *Nature*, 342: 115.

BOULTER, D., GATEHOUSE, J. A., GATEHOUSE, A. M. R., *et al.* (1990), 'Genetic engineering of plants for insect resistance', *Endeavour*, 14: 185.

BRAHAMS, D. (1990), 'Human genetic information: the legal implications', in D. Chadwick *et al.* (eds.) (1990), *Human Genetic Information: Science, Law and Ethics*, J. Wiley & Sons, p. 117.

BRENNER, S. (1989), *Molecular Biology—A Selection of Papers*, Academic Press.

BROBERG, O., *et al.* (1990), Technical University of Denmark, personal communication.

CAREY, N. H., and CRAWLEY, P. E., 'Commercial exploitation of the human genome: what are the problems', in D. Chadwick *et al.* (eds.) (1990), *Human Genetic Information: Science, Law and Ethics*, J. Wiley & Sons, pp. 141–2.

CHERFAS, J. (1982), *Man Made Life—A Genetic Engineering Primer*, Basil Blackwell.

CLARK, A. J., SIMONS, P., WILMUT, I., *et al.* (1987), 'Pharmaceuticals from transgenic livestock', *Trends in Biotechnology*, 5: 20.

CLARKE, C. A. (1987), *Human Genetics and Medicine* (3rd edn.), Edward Arnold.

Committee of the Health Council of the Netherlands (1989),

Heredity Science and Society, The Health Council of the Netherlands.

COUTELLE, C., WILLIAMS, C., HANDYSIDE, A., et al. (1989), 'Genetic analysis of DNA from single human oocytes: a model for preimplantation diagnosis of cystic fibrosis', *British Medical Journal*, 299: 22.

DARNELL, J., LODISH, H., and BALTIMORE, D. (1986), *Molecular Cell Biology*, Scientific American Books.

DAVIES, K., and GERSHON, D. (1990), 'Law to keep labels off genes', *Nature*, 347: 221.

DELANNAY, X., LaVALLEE, B. J., PROKSCH, R. K., et al. (1989), 'Field performance of transgenic tomato plants expressing the *Bacillus thuringiensis* var, *Kurstaki* insect control protein', *Bio/Technology*, 7: 1265.

DICKSON, D. (1985), 'A push for European patent reform', *Science* (24 May), 926–7.

DIXON, B. (1988), *Engineered Organisms in the Environment*, Regem Ltd.

EC Commission (1986), *Council Directive for the Protection of Animals Used for Experimental and Other Scientific Purposes*, 86/609/EEC.

—— (1989), *Proposal for a Council Directive on the Legal Protection of Biotechnological Inventions*, COM(88)496 final.

—— (1990), *Draft Proposal for a Council Regulation Concerning the Use of Certain Substances and Techniques Intended for Administration or Application to Animals to Stimulate their Productivity*, Document VI/3670/90-Rev.1.

EISENSTEIN, B. I. (1990), 'The polymerase chain reaction', *New England Journal of Medicine*, 322: 178.

ERSLEV, A. J. (1991), 'Erythropoietin', *New England Journal of Medicine*, 324: 1339.

EVANS, R. M. (1988), 'The steroid and thyroid hormone receptor superfamily', *Science*, 240: 889–95.

FINCHAM, J. R. S., and RAVETZ, J. R. (1991), *Genetically Engineered Organisms*, Open University Press.

FRADKIN, J. E., SCHONBERGER, L. B., MILLS, J. L., et al. (1991), 'Creutzfeldt-Jacob disease in pituitary growth hormone recipients in the United states', *Journal of the American Medical Association*, 265: 880.

FREELAND JUDSON, H. (1979), *The Eighth Day of Creation—the Makers of the Revolution in Biology*, Jonathan Cape.

FRIEDMAN, O., quoted in McKie, R. (1988), *The Genetic Jigsaw*, Oxford University Press.

GOODMAN, B. (1990), 'The genetic anatomy of us (and a few friends)', *BioScience*, 40: 484.

GRAHAM, A., PAPALOPOULU, N., and KRUMLAUF, R. (1989), 'The murine and *Drosophila* homeobox gene complexes have common features of organization and expression', *Cell*, 57: 367–78.

HAMPTON, M. L., ANDERSON, J., LAVIZZO, B. S., and BERGMAN, A. B. (1974), 'Sickle cell "non-disease"', *American Journal of Childhood Diseases*, 128: 58–61.

HANDYSIDE, A. H., KONTAGIANNI, E. H., HARDY, K., and WINSTON, R. M. (1990), 'Pregnancies from biopsied human preimplantation embryos sexed by Y-specific DNA amplification', *Nature*, 344: 768.

HIATT, A., CAFFERKEY, R., and BOWDISH, K. (1989), 'Production of antibodies in transgenic plants', *Nature*, 342: 76.

HOLDING, C., and MONK, M. (1989), 'Diagnosis of beta-thalassaemia by DNA amplification in single blastomeres from mouse preimplantation embryos', *Lancet*, 2: 532.

HOPWOOD, D. A. (1989), 'Antibiotics: opportunities for genetic manipulation', *Phil. Trans. R. Soc. Lond. B*. 324: 549.

JAENISCH, R. (1988), 'Transgenic animals', *Science*, 240: 1468.

KING, D. (1991), 'The Ultimate Claim', *Chemistry and Industry* (3 June), 404.

LEVIDOW, L., and TAIT, J. (1990), 'The Greening of Biotechnology: From GMOs to Environmentally-Friendly Products', Open University Occasional Paper, p. 12, and *Science and Public Policy*, forthcoming.

LEWIN, B. (1990), *Genes IV*, Oxford University Press.

LINDSEY, K., and JONES, M. G. K. (1989), *Plant Biotechnology in Agriculture*, Open University Press.

LUZIO, J. P., and THOMPSON, R. J. (1990), *Molecular Medical Biochemistry*, Cambridge University Press.

McKIE, R. (1988), *The Genetic Jigsaw*, Oxford University Press.

MACKLIN, R. (1985), 'Mapping the Human Genome: Problems of Privacy and Free Choice', in A. Milansky and G. J. Annas (eds.) (1985), *Genetics and the Law III*, Plenum Press, ch. 10.

McNEIL, M., *et al.* (1990), *The New Reproductive Technologies*, Macmillan.

MARX, J. L. (ed.) (1989), *A Revolution in Biotechnology*, Cambridge University Press.

MODELL, M., and MODELL, B. (1990), 'Genetic screening for ethnic minorities', *British Medical Journal*, 300: 1702.

MONK, M., HANDYSIDE, A., HARDY, K., and WHITTINGHAM, D. (1987), 'Preimplantation diagnosis of deficiency of hypoxanthine phosphoribosyl transferase in a mouse model for Lesch-Nyhan syndrome', *Lancet*, 2: 426.

—— and HOLDING, C. (1990), 'Amplification of a beta haemoglobin sequence in individual human oocytes and polar bodies', *Lancet*, 335: 988.

MOONEY, H. A., and BERNARDI, G. (1990), *Introduction of Genetically Modified Organisms into the Environment*, Wiley.

MORONE, J. G., and WOODHOUSE, E. J. (1986), *Averting Catastrophe*, University of California Press.

MOTULSKY, A. G. (1983), 'Impact of Genetic Manipulation on Society and Medicine', *Science*, 219: 135–40.

MULLIS, K. B. (1990), 'The unusual origin of the polymerase chain reaction', *Scientific American* (Apr.), 36.

NIH Technology Assessment Panel (1991), 'Conference statement on bovine somatotropin', *Journal of the American Medical Association*, 265: 1423.

NOSSAL, G. J. V., and COPPEL, R. L. (1989), *Reshaping Life* (2nd edn.), Cambridge University Press.

OECD (1986), *Recombinant DNA Safety Considerations*.

OLD, J. M., THEIN, S. L., WEATHERALL, D. J., *et al.* (1989), 'Pre-natal diagnosis of the major haemoglobin disorders', *Mol. Biol. Med.* 6: 55.

OLSON, E. N. (1990), 'MyoD family: a paradigm for development?', *Genes and Development*, 4: 1454–61.

POTRYKUS, I. (1990), 'Gene transfer to cereals: an assessment', *Bio/Technology*, 8: 535.

PURSEL, V. G., PINKERT, C. A., MILLER, K. F., *et al.* (1989), 'Genetic engineering of livestock', *Science*, 244: 1281.

RAVETZ, J. (1990), *The Merger of Power with Knowledge*, Mansell Publishing Ltd.

REDFERN, M. (1990), *Transgenesis in Animals—A Briefing Document*, Royal Society.

REILLY, P. R. (1991), 'Advantages of genetic testing outweigh arguments against widespread screening', *Scientist* (21 Jan.), 9.

ROBERTS, L. (1987), 'Who owns the human genome?', *Science*, 237: 336.

ROSENBERG, S. A., AEBERSOLD, P., CORNETTA, K., *et al.* (1990), 'Gene transfer to humans—immunotherapy of patients with advanced melanoma, using tumor-infiltrating lymphocytes modified by retroviral gene transduction', *New England Journal of Medicine*, 323: 570.

ROSENFIELD, I., ZIFF, E., and VAN LOON, B. (1983), *DNA for Beginners*, Norton.

Royal College of Physicians of London (1990), *Teaching Genetics to Medical Students: A Survey and Recommendations.*

Royal Commission on Environmental Pollution (1989), *The Release of Genetically Engineered Organisms to the Environment*, 13th Report, HMSO.

RUSSELL, P. J. (1987), *Essential Genetics* (2nd edn.), Blackwell Scientific Publications.

SAPIENZA, C. (1990), 'Parental imprinting of genes', *Scientific American* (Oct.), 26.

SEIDEL, G. E. (1989), 'Geneticists in the pasture', *Technology Review* (Apr.), 43.

SHACKLEY, S. J. (1989), 'Regulation of the release of genetically manipulated organisms into the environment', *Science and Public Policy*, 16: 211.

SIMONS, J. P., WILMUT, I., CLARK, A. J., *et al.* (1988), 'Gene transfer into sheep', *Bio/Technology*, 6: 179.

SLACK, J. M. W. (1991), *From Egg to Embryo* (2nd edn.), Cambridge University Press.

STAMATOYANNOPOULOS, G. (1974), 'Problems of screening and counselling in the meoglobinopathies', in A. G. Motulsky, W. Lenz, and F. J. G. Ebling (eds.) (1974), *Birth Defects: Proceedings of the 4th International Conference*, Excerpta Medica, pp. 269–74.

STEPHENS, J. C., CAVANAUGH, M. L., GRADIE, M. I., *et al.* (1990), 'Mapping the human genome: current status', *Science*, 250: 237.

STRAUGHAN R. (1989), *The Genetic Manipulation of Plants, Animals and Microbes*, National Consumer Council.

STURTEVANT, A. H. (1965), *A History of Genetics*, Harper & Row.

SUSSMAN, M., COLLINS, C. H., SKINNER, F. A., and STEWART-TULL, D. E. (1988), *The Release of Genetically-Engineered Micro-Organisms*, Academic Press.

SUZUKI, D., and KNUDTSON, P. (1990), *Genethics: The Ethics of Engineering Life*, Unwin Hyman.

TIEDJE, J. M., COLWELL, R. K., GROSSMAN, Y. L., *et al.* (1989), 'The planned introduction of genetically engineered organisms: ecological considerations and recommendations', *Ecology*, 70: 298–315.

US Office of Technology Assessment (1988), *New Developments in Biotechnology—Field-Testing Engineered Organisms*, OTA.

VERMA, I. M. (1990), 'Gene therapy', *Scientific American* (Nov.), 34.

WALDEN, R. (1988), *Genetic Transformation in Plants*, Open University Press.

WAMBAUGH, J. (1990), *The Blooding*, Bantam Books.

WATSON, J. D. (1990), 'The human genome project: past, present and future', *Science*, 248: 44.

—— HOPKINS, N. H., ROBERTS, J. W., STEITZ, J. A., and WEINER, A. M. (1987), *Molecular Biology of the Gene* (4th edn.), Benjamin Cummins Publishing Co.

—— and TOOZE, J. (1981), *The DNA Story*, Freeman.

WATTS, S. (1991), 'A matter of life and patents', *New Scientist* (12 Jan.), 57.

WEATHERALL, D. J. (1985), *The New Genetics and Clinical Practice* (2nd edn.), Oxford University Press.

—— (1991), 'Gene therapy in perspective', *Nature*, 349 (24 Jan.), 275.

WHEALE, P., and McNALLY, R. (1988), *Genetic Engineering: Catastrophe or Utopia?*, Wheatsheaf.

WHITE, R., and LALOUEL, J.-M. (1988), 'Chromosome mapping with DNA markers', *Scientific American* (Feb.), 40.

WILLIAMSON, M., PERRINS, J., and FITTER, A. (1990), 'Releasing genetically engineered plants—present proposals and possible hazards', *Trends in Ecology and Evolution*, 5: 417.

WINTER, G., and MILSTEIN, C. (1991), 'Man-made antibodies', *Nature*, 349: 293.

WINTER, G. P. (1989), 'Antibody engineering', *Phil. Trans. R. Soc. Lond. B*. 324: 537.

WITT, S. C. (1990), *Biotechnology, Microbes and the Environment*, Center for Science Information.

GLOSSARY

allele. One of a number of alternative forms of a gene or DNA sequence occurring at the same position on each homologous chromosome.

amino acid. The building blocks of protein. 20 different amino acids are generally found in proteins though several hundred are known.

amniocentesis. A procedure whereby amniotic fluid is taken through a needle from the amniotic cavity. The fluid and the cells that it contains can then be analysed to determine genetic abnormalities in the fetus.

antibody. A protein synthesized by the immune system in response to the presence of a specific foreign antigen.

anticodon. A sequence of three consecutive bases in tRNA which binds with a complementary mRNA codon.

antigen. A substance that stimulates the immune system to produce specific antibodies against it.

bacteria. Large group of typically single-cell micro-organisms, most of which are parasites.

bacteriophage. A virus that infects bacterial cells.

chimaera. A human or animal in which two or more different cell lines co-exist, coming from more than two gametes. Chimaeras can occur naturally when the two halves of an egg are fertilized by different sperm or artificially by mixing cells of two distinct organisms.

chorionic villus sampling (CVS). A procedure whereby cells are taken from the developing placenta using a needle guided by ultrasound. The cells share the genetic make-up of the fetus and can be analysed for genetic abnormalities.

chromatid. One of the two identical strands in a replicating chromosome during mitosis or meiosis.

chromosome. A threadlike structure, found in the nuclei of cells, which contains genes in linear sequence. Humans have 23 pairs of chromosomes.

clone. Genetically identical cells or organisms arising from mitotic division of a single cell.

codon. Sequence of three consecutive bases in mRNA coding for an amino acid.

conjugation. Process by which genetic material is transferred from one organism to another during cell-to-cell contact.

crossover. Exchange of segments of DNA between homologous chromatids during meiosis.

differentiation. Process of specialization of cells into tissues and organs.

dimer. Compound comprised of two molecules.

diploid. A cell containing two sets of chromosomes. Most cells apart from the sex cells are diploid.

DNA (deoxyribonucleic acid). The primary genetic material of all cells. DNA contains a backbone of sugar (deoxyribose) and phosphate molecules to which are attached, along its length and in any order, four different substances known as bases.

DNA ligase. An enzyme that joins nucleotides in a DNA strand.

dominant. Trait expressed in a person who is heterozygous for a particular gene (cf. recessive).

electrophoresis. A technique for separating different sized fragments of DNA based on their variable mobility in an electric field. Small fragments migrate faster than large fragments in the field.

enzyme. A protein that acts as a biological catalyst.

eugenics. The study of methods of improving the quality of the human race especially by selective breeding.

eukaryote. An organism whose cells contain a true nucleus and which undergo mitosis.

exon. Stretches of DNA in a gene which code for protein product after the intervening, non-coding sequences (introns) have been spliced out.

gamete. A haploid sex cell, such as a spermatozoon or ovum.

gene. A stretch of DNA, occupying a fixed position on a chromosome, which specifies the production of a protein or part of a protein.

gene therapy. The replacement or repair of defective genes in living cells.

genome. The total genetic content of a gamete.

genotype. The genetic constitution of an individual organism or person.

germ cells. The cells from which sperm and ova develop.

haemoglobin. Protein in red blood cells which is responsible for transporting oxygen to the tissues.

haploid. A cell containing one set of chromosomes. All gametes (sperm and ova) are haploid.

heterozygous. Having two different alleles at a particular locus on homologous chromosomes.

homozygous. Having two identical alleles at a particular locus on homologous chromosomes.

hybrid. An offspring of a cross between two genetically dissimilar individuals.

intron. The non-coding sequences in genes which are read during transcription but spliced out before translation into protein product.

linkage. Two or more alleles situated close together on the same chromosome which tend to be inherited together.

locus. Site of a specific gene or DNA sequence on a chromosome.

marker. General term for a DNA sequence, frequently a polymorphism, which occurs close to a gene and which is used to track the gene. It can be used, similarly, to track organisms.

meiosis. Cell division during the formation of gametes that reduces the number of chromosomes in each cell to one half (haploid) and allows the exchange of segments of DNA between homologous chromatids.

messenger RNA (mRNA). An RNA molecule, produced from DNA during transcription, which carries genetic information to ribosomes where it is translated into an amino acid sequence.

microbe. Any microscopic infective agent, especially a disease-causing bacterium.

mitosis. Cell division following replication of the chromosomes resulting in diploid daughter cells identical to the parent cell.

monogenic. Controlled by or associated with a single gene.

mosaic. Presence in a person of two different cell lines derived from a single zygote.

multifactorial. Controlled by or associated with many genes plus the effects of the environment.

mutation. Alteration in the structure of DNA or RNA.

nucleotide. Subunit of a nucleic acid composed of a sugar, phosphate, and one of the bases adenine, cytosine, guanine, thymine, or uracil.

oncogene. A gene with the potential to cause cancer.

operon. A group of adjacent structural genes together with the regions which control their transcription into a single mRNA.

phenotype. The observable characteristics of an individual as determined by the interaction of its genetic constitution and the environment in which development occurs.

plasmid. A small circular piece of DNA found in some bacteria which replicates independently of the main bacterial DNA.

polygenic. Controlled by or associated with more than one gene.

polymerase chain reaction (PCR). Laboratory process by which a specific DNA sequence is copied many times in only a few hours to enable subsequent analysis of the DNA.

polymorphism. The presence of several common forms of a genetic characteristic in a population.

prion. Small infectious particles of protein found in brain tissue of humans and other species suffering from spongiform encephalopathy e.g. Creutzfeldt-Jacob disease.

probe. A stretch of radioactively labelled DNA used to detect RNA or complementary sequences in a DNA sample.

prokaryote. An organism that lacks a true nucleus, e.g. bacteria, and does not undergo mitosis.

recessive. Trait expressed in people who are homozygous for a particular gene but not in those who are heterozygous for the gene.

recombinant DNA (rDNA). A new DNA sequence produced artificially by joining pieces of foreign DNA together.

recombination. Crossing over of genetic material between homologous chromosomes during meiosis resulting in a new combination of alleles on each chromosome.

restriction endonuclease. Enzyme that cuts double-stranded DNA at a specific nucleotide sequence to produce restriction fragments.

restriction fragment length polymorphism (RFLP). Inherited variations in the size of DNA fragments produced when DNA is cut with a specific restriction endonuclease.

retrovirus. An RNA virus that replicates itself by making a complementary DNA molecule upon infecting cells.

reverse transcriptase. The enzyme used by retroviruses to synthesize DNA from its RNA template.

RNA (ribonucleic acid). Genetic material present in all living cells essential for the synthesis of proteins. Unlike DNA it is single-stranded, and has the sugar ribose instead of deoxyribose and the base uracil instead of thymine.

somatic cells. All body cells except the gametes and the cells from which they derive.

stem cell. Undifferentiated cell which gives rise to specialized cells such as blood cells.

transcription. Production of messenger RNA from a DNA sequence in a gene.

transfer RNA (tRNA). The RNA involved in translating the coded information in mRNA into protein. Each tRNA molecule carries a single amino acid and has three specific bases (anticodon) which are complementary to the corresponding bases in mRNA which code for that amino acid.

transgenic. The term used to describe organisms which have been altered to carry and express genes from another species.

translation. Production of protein from messenger RNA.

vector. The plasmid, virus, or other vehicle used to carry a cloned DNA sequence into the cell of another species.

virus. Microbe consisting of a DNA or (RNA) core, surrounded by protein, which can only replicate in the cells of a host organism.

X-linked. Term used to describe genes carried on the X chromosome.

INDEX

Note: all entries refer to genes or genetics unless otherwise stated